Latino Gay [

Latino Gay Men and HIV

Culture, Sexuality, and Risk Behavior

Rafael M. Díaz

ROUTLEDGE
New York and London

Published in 1998 by
Routledge
29 West 35th Street
New York, NY 10001

Published in Great Britain in 1998 by
Routledge
11 New Fetter Lane
London EC4P 4EE

Printed in the United States of America on acid-free paper
Design: Jack Donner

Library of Congress Cataloging-in-Publication Data

Díaz, Rafael M., 1950–
Latino gay men and HIV: culture, sexuality, and risk behavior / Rafael M. Díaz.
     p.   cm.
  Includes index.
  ISBN 0–415–91387–X (hardcover). — 0–415–91388–8 (pbk.)
  1. AIDS (Disease)—United States—Prevention.   2. Hispanic American gays—Diseases.   I. Title.
RA644.A25D53   1998
362.1'969792'008968073—dc21   97–23167
                                                                  CIP

To Jeffrey Moulton Benevedes and Barbara VanOss Marín,
for their loving support in difficult moments of transition.
And to Michael Vincent Domínguez, for being there when I arrived.

In loving memory of my colleague and friend,
Reinaldo Ortiz-Colón (1950–1996)

Contents

Acknowledgments

My life is blessed with a great deal of support from family, colleagues, and friends. I am well aware that the fruits of my work, especially manuscripts that I sign and take credit for, are not mine alone, but more properly are the fruits of social collaboration at many different levels, personal and professional.

I want to thank first my colleagues and friends at the Center for AIDS Prevention Studies (CAPS) at the University of California San Francisco (UCSF). Under the leadership of our director, Thomas J. Coates, who is one of the most suppportive mentors I've ever had, CAPS has given me a nurturing, stimulating, and challenging context in which to formulate and develop the research and ideas presented in this book. Even though sometimes I speak with force about matters that I don't understand much, CAPS colleagues have listened attentively, as well as read and reviewed my work with deep respect and genuine enthusiasm. At CAPS, I received the post-doctoral training and the personal encouragement I needed to make a difficult transition into a new field of research. In particular, my colleague and friend Barbara V. Marín went well beyond the call of duty to nurture my emerging career as an HIV prevention researcher. Her contributions to my work are many, ranging from financial support to compensate research participants to last-minute detailed reviews of my written work and, more importantly, a good shoulder to cry on when the data touched deep places of personal vulnerability. I am quite fortunate to work in such a supportive environment and am grateful to the funding sources that make CAPS and my work possible, in particular, the National Institute of Mental Health and the National Institute of Child Health and Human Development.

The research presented in this book, including extensive interviews with Latino gay men, was made possible through the enthusiastic collaboration with many individuals and organizations that tirelessly service this population. I am indebted to Victor Gaitán for providing access to a world of Latino gay culture I was barely familiar with, and to colleagues at the Mission Neighborhood Health Center (MNHC) who helped me put to the test some of my ideas through practical applications. At MNHC I have been blessed with the support of terrific and highly committed individuals such as Brenda Storey, Ricardo Newball, Rómulo Hernández, and José Ramón Fernández-Peña. Through the project El Ambiente, and in collaboration with Eduardo Morales, Eugene Dilán, and Richard Rodríguez, I was able to collect valuable data and explore new avenues for HIV prevention with Latino gay men. The National Latino/a Lesbian and Gay Organization (LLEGO) and, in particular, Martín Ornelas-Quintero and Robert Vázquez were instrumental in supporting and revising the literature review included in the book; their perspectives as community members and activists helped me stay close to the voices of the men about whom I was writing.

I am also indebted to the San Francisco AIDS Foundation (SFAF) for inviting me to participate and analyze data collected in their innovative Qualitative Interview Study (QIS). Through the SFAF/QIS study, I was able to work with and receive valuable feedback from individuals who are at the forefront of HIV prevention research and practice. With the risk of missing some important names, I want to thank members of the QIS project, in particular René Durazzo, Ron Stall, Andy Williams, and Michael Crosby for their collegial support in the context of this project.

This book project began with the enthusiastic encouragement and support of Philip Rappaport, formerly psychology editor at Routledge. His successor, Heidi Freund, has provided the needed encouragement to bring the project to completion. Also, many details associated with the final stages of manuscript preparation for publication were done by Miguel Casuso, Project Coordinator of the Latino Gay Men Study at CAPS. Without Miguel's hard work and attention to detail, I am afraid the project would not have been completed in a timely fashion.

I want to thank family and friends who have supported me in so many different ways. My parents Zaida and Rafael who, even though pained about their son's homosexuality, have conveyed the clear message that, above all, I am their son and I'll always be supported and welcome by them. I also want to acknowledge the support of my sister Zaida and my cousin Nelia with whom I can talk openly about my life; through their support, I have been able to integrate aspects of my life that would be otherwise painfully disjointed.

Last, but not least, I want to thank all the Latino gay men who participated in the research reported in this book. They offered me their time, their voices, and their heart-felt experiences, at times taking the risk of breaking years of silence about matters most important to them. Their voices literally fill many pages of this book. In many important ways, they are the real authors; I hope they see the book as a worthy and truthful channel.

Preface

As we enter the sixteenth year of the tragic HIV epidemic in our midst—frustrated, angry, and tired with multiple loss and grief—we, Latino gay men, are called to a period of deep reflection, critical thinking, and self-observation. Passionate more than ever to stop the spread of HIV among our lovers, brothers, and friends, we must examine what we know, listen to the voices of those most seriously affected, and examine the most promising attempts to intervene. Only then can we undertake with renewed vigor our most intelligent preventive actions.

With few exceptions, HIV risk-reduction interventions to date have not been successful in significantly decreasing, much less stopping, the spread of HIV among Latino gay men in the U.S. As of today, there are no published reports of scientifically evaluated HIV prevention programs directed specifically at this community. Painfully lacking in the literature are the voices and subjective experiences of Latino gay men, as we struggle to remain healthy and live fulfilling sexual lives in the midst of a devastating epidemic.

Though limited in both number and scope, the epidemiological and behavioral research literature does contain a number of important research studies that shed light on our difficult situation. There are also several innovative attempts, not yet formally evaluated, to reduce the risk of HIV transmission among Latino gay men in a culturally appropriate manner. Carefully considered, the findings of these studies and the experiences of these innovative projects may open new avenues for effective AIDS education and prevention and, more importantly, hope.

This book was thus written to review the epidemiological and behavioral literature, to bring the voices of Latino gay men to the work of HIV prevention, and to present an integrating picture of the psychological and cultural context in which the virus is spreading at seemingly explosive rates. In part, the book is written as a guide for all those individuals who have responsibility for designing, implementing, and evaluating HIV prevention interventions for this highly affected community. It is also meant as a tool for critical reflection and self-observation for the empowerment of Latino gay men in their day-to-day struggle with a fatal sexually transmitted disease. Above all, the book has been written to provide meaning rather than convey blame in a very difficult, high-risk situation.

In the fall of 1994, as I was beginning work on this book, I attended the conference on Gay Men of Color and AIDS in Chicago, sponsored by the National Task Force on AIDS Prevention. In the conference I joined approximately 200 hundred gay men of color who are in charge of designing and implementing HIV risk-reduction programs for their communities across the nation. The conference brought together the world of HIV prevention services, a world of men and women working incredibly hard in the trenches, at both the local and national levels, to stop this epidemic.

This world of prevention workers, however, seemed so very different, separated and untouched by my world of behavioral research, by my meetings at the National Institutes of Health, by the post-doctoral seminars and the peer-review sessions at my research center! As one of the few researchers in the Chicago audience, I acutely experienced the overwhelming gap between the world of research and the world of prevention. I became keenly aware that if we want to stop this epidemic we must somehow bring these two separate worlds together. Specifically, we must calibrate the research enterprise with the needs and questions of HIV prevention practitioners.

In Chicago, I wondered how many Latino gay men who design and run HIV prevention programs—those who are indeed my most precious audience—did read my latest research manuscript on Latino gay men in the Southwestern United States (Díaz, Stall, Hoff, Daigle, and Coates, 1996). Would they be turned off by the research style of writing? Would they know what the findings of multivariate analyses meant? Would they know how to incorporate the findings into their busy and exhausting world of HIV prevention services? I have written this book with these questions in mind, knowing quite well that the value of this effortful enterprise depends on the book's ability to bridge the worlds of research and practice. I ask for readers' help in such an enormous undertaking.

In fact, my dream is that this book is not only read, studied, and critically discussed, but also put to good use by all those who work in community-based and government organizations aimed at HIV prevention with Latino gay men. In the field of HIV prevention, research findings and theoretical statements are valuable to the extent that they lead to interventions that are measurably effective. The validity of our knowledge lies ultimately in its usefulness to guide and promote desired change. Thus, it is up to workers in the challenging world of HIV prevention to demonstrate the validity of the research findings and theoretical statements presented in this book.

Introduction

"We Now Have the Knowledge . . ."
Do We?

Every new HIV infection is a needless infection. . . . We now have the
knowledge and technology to prevent the sexual spread of HIV.

—Donna Shalala, U.S. Secretary
of Health and Human Services, January 1994

As we move through the second decade of the AIDS epidemic, well-
equipped with both "knowledge and technology" to avoid further
infection, it is disheartening to witness the increasing spread of HIV
among vulnerable groups—minority women, adolescents, gay men of
color. For me, a 46-year-old Latino gay man living in San Francisco,
the situation is particularly trying. Almost on a daily basis, I see rising
curves in epidemiological charts and witness the thinning and yellow-
ing faces of AIDS among lovers, friends, and other members of my
community. It is painfully obvious that "knowledge" (about modes of
HIV transmission and means of prevention) and "technology" (with
assumed reference to the availability of latex condoms, nonoxynol-9,
and the mass media to promote them), though necessary, are not suffi-
cient to stop the spread of this devastating disease.

Knowledge-Behavior Inconsistency

There is plenty of evidence, reviewed with greater detail in Chapter 2,
documenting that Latino gay men possess a relatively high level of

knowledge about the modes of HIV transmission and the effective means of prevention. For example, in a recent study of gay men in five southern states (Alabama, Florida, Lousiana, North Carolina, and Texas), sponsored by the National Task Force in AIDS Prevention, Latinos responded quite accurately to difficult items that assessed information about condoms: the effectiveness of latex over lambskin (78% correct) and the protection utility of nonoxynol-9 (83% correct). In addition, Latino gay men were accurate in identifying that withdrawal before ejaculation does not prevent transmission (82% correct), that the inserter "top" partner in unprotected anal intercourse is also at risk (83% correct), and that it is not possible to tell by appearances alone whether a sex partner has AIDS (85% correct).

The fact that such high and sophisticated levels of knowledge about HIV transmission exist in cities not considered AIDS epicenters is definitely impressive and supports Secretary Shalala's optimistic remarks. However, a large proportion (37%) of these knowledgeable men in the South also reported practicing unprotected anal intercourse at least once during the thirty days before the survey interview. Other surveys of Latino gay men in the U.S. converge on similar findings. With estimates ranging from about 30% to 50% of different samples, and in the presence of both substantial knowledge and relatively strong intentions to practice safer sex, Latino gay men still engage in unprotected anal intercourse, a practice that constitutes one of the most efficient routes for HIV transmission.

For quite some time now, psychologists have known that knowledge, as well as other "cognitive" variables, are poor predictors of behavior. Knowledge and attitudes might be important predictors of behavioral intentions; however, the effective *enactment* of those intentions is complicated by a host of contextual and psychosocial factors that compete with or weaken self-formulated plans of action. This is clear to most of us when we review the fate of our new year's resolutions regarding diet, exercise, or increased personal organization. It definitely takes more than knowledge to act effectively in an intentional, self-determined way. This is especially true within the complex domain of human sexuality.

I began my investigations of Latino gay men and HIV approximately five years ago, in the fall of 1992. Focusing on the documented disconnection between HIV knowledge and risky sexual behavior, I interviewed approximately 70 men in the contexts of focus groups and individual interviews. I wanted to understand the subjective experience of Latino gay men in San Francisco as they struggled to maintain or surrendered the practice of safer sex. Among the men I interviewed, subjective reactions to the knowledge-behavior inconsistency varied from fatalism—"We know we are going to get it [HIV] sooner or later"—to blatant self-deprecation—"Face it, girl, we think with our crotches."

I quickly learned that Latino gay men who practice risky behavior, for the most part, are well aware of their incongruent behavior and of the serious risk their unprotected behavior represents. However, it seems to me that there is a major lack of understanding about *why* this is the case. While they know intricate details about the virus and how it is transmitted, and what is needed for protection, Latino gay men seemed to know very little about themselves as sexual beings, with little self-awareness of what threatens their sense of sexual control or the situations and circumstances that undermine their safer sex intentions. I have no doubts that the majority of these men want to be safe and remain healthy—many begin their Friday evenings and initiate sexual encounters with relatively strong safer sex intentions and condoms in their pockets—but they also helplessly confess their surrender to passion and their inability to enact their intentions and remain safe in emotionally and sexually charged situations. When asked about it, many men responded, "I don't know." Not surprisingly, the situation breeds further fatalism, helplessness, self-deprecation, and, of course, HIV infection.

Reasons for the Inconsistency

Even though an inconsistent relation between knowledge and behavior is by no means unique to Latino gay men, I believe that the reasons for the particular inconsistency must be found in our unique sociocultural and psychosocial situations, in the unique ways that we perceive ourselves and our sexuality and give meaning to our world. It is precisely these contextual, cultural, and psychosocial variables affecting the lives of Latino gay men that must be investigated in order to understand and intervene with the observed AIDS knowledge-intention-behavior disparity. A major aim of this book is to share my investigation of the sociocultural variables that compete with the enactment of safer sex intentions among Latino gay men.

As Latino gay men, we must ultimately take responsibility for our own actions. However, I want to propose that our safer sex intentions are too often weakened by strong factors in our culture such as machismo, homophobia, poverty, racism, and sexual silence, to name a few. These factors are larger or greater than the individuals who intend to perform a given behavior. These factors, however, are no longer outside of ourselves; they are socializing and oppressive forces that have become internalized in our sexual development. It is my belief that these cultural values and socialization forces have not only shaped but also currently regulate our sexuality, competing against self-formulated plans of action regarding safer sex.

For example, a strong machismo discourse, widely diffused within the socialization practices of many Latino families, does associate masculinity with risk taking, low sexual control, and sexual prowess with multiple partners. For Latino boys, machismo is further ingrained by the message that manhood is neither biologically given nor environmentally acquired, but rather must be "proven" from an early age with "macho acts" congruent with the culture's definition of masculinity. Because sexual penetration is a favored and well-defined act to prove masculinity, it is no surprise that many Latino men have difficulties adopting non-penetrative sex practices or risking the loss of an erection by wearing condoms. Risky sexual behavior among men socialized within Latino communities must be understood in the context of these internalized messages. These messages, now fully internalized and integrated in our views of self and the world, constitute major barriers to safer sex practices.

Unfortunately, these sociocultural messages and the barriers they create, with very few exceptions, have been virtually ignored by education, prevention, and research programs. Moreover, I would venture to say that the spread of HIV in my community has actually been facilitated by poorly developed prevention efforts and by a slim body of research that keeps us in the dark with respect to the subjective experiences of Latino gay men and our struggles within the epidemic. Thus, I would like to devote a major part of this introductory chapter to offering a critical review of current prevention and education efforts and research to date, not in the spirit of blame—I do indeed want to pay respect to those who have worked and are working so very hard to stop AIDS in my community through both direct services and research—but in the spirit of learning the lessons to be learned, becoming a bit wiser, and exploring new avenues for more effective interventions and more enlightening research.

Three Limitations of Current Interventions

At the risk of over-generalizing, I would like to propose that, at present, the majority of AIDS risk-reduction interventions directed at Latino gay men suffer from three important shortcomings. First, they tend to be directed at "men who have sex with men" (MSM), rather than at self-identified gay/bisexual men. Second, they are implemented within a "deficit" pedagogy, where risky sexual behavior is seen as a lack (or deficit) of knowledge, motivation, and skill. Finally, interventions rarely take notice that (so-called) risky sexual behavior is not only natural but also *meaningful* behavior, and that its occurrence, with full awareness of the risk involved, can be quite logical and congruent from a given sociocultural perspective. Let us examine these limitations of HIV risk-reduction interventions in some detail.

The Problem with MSM

In the name of cultural sensitivity and "political correctness," health practitioners and educators have favored the term "men who have sex with men" (MSM) when describing the population of men who engage in same-sex behavior, especially if these men are from ethnic and racial minorities. According to its proponents, there are three distinct advantages in using the term MSM. First, the label accurately recognizes that same-sex behavior can occur without impacting an individual's self-identification as heterosexual. It is widely recognized that, among many heterosexually identified Latinos, insertive anal intercourse on other men is not labeled as homosexual, and it can occur without questioning or threatening the individual's heterosexual orientation. A second advantage is that the proponents of the MSM label accurately recognize that the label "gay" may be charged with cultural connotations applicable only to men who are out to family, friends, and co-workers, and who both participate in and identify as members of a mainstream (mostly White, middle class) gay community. These characteristics associated with a gay identity in the U.S. might not be true of targeted individuals, especially if they are men of color who have enormous difficulties being "out" within their own families and minority communities, and who might feel left out or out of place within the mainstream gay community for reasons of race, social class, or both. Finally, because in this population the transmission of HIV occurs mostly through unprotected anal intercourse, and the virus does not make distinctions regarding self-identified sexual orientation, the MSM label is seen as inclusive of those at risk for practicing the risk behavior—homosexual, gay, bisexual, transgender, and straight men who have unprotected sex with other men—regardless of self-identification. Thus, it is not surprising that the term MSM has been welcome by all those dealing with the diversity and complexity of same-sex behavior in Latino communities, practitioners and researchers alike.

Nonetheless, I would like to argue that there are some serious problems and disadvantages in considering MSM as the client population, especially in risk-reduction programs that actually serve or are supposed to target Latinos who do indeed self-identify as homosexual or gay. First of all, there are substantial differences between gay-identified men and heterosexually identified MSM on variables relevant to AIDS education and prevention. For one, the emotional impact and subjective meaning of same-sex behavior—the very same behavior targeted for change—sets the two groups worlds apart. For gay or homosexually identified men, same-sex acts often occur in the context of lover or potential lover relationships, within a romantic and emotional context where issues of acceptance and rejection, the individual's self-esteem, and the need for love and social connection are paramount. In fact, those emotional, romantic, and personal needs will determine to a great extent whether protection in sexual encounters will be negotiated or even talked about (Kelly et al., 1991). For example, fear of rejection by a desirable potential lover might keep men silent about issues regarding HIV and the need for protection.

Lumping self-identified gay men with other MSM does not take into account the complex personal dilemmas and serious social consequences of homosexual self-identification within Latino communities. For many of these men, "coming out" to themselves and others is a painful process that involves the risk of social isolation, economic hardship, or both. Of crucial importance is the fact that, for the majority of

Latino men, self-identification as homosexual presents an enormous challenge to the relationship with family members, many of whom see homosexuality as a source of shame and dishonor for the whole family.

It is widely recognized that close and supportive family relations hold an important place for Latinos throughout the life span. In this country, family supportive relations among Latinos are seen as the main protective factor against the stresses of poverty and minority status. For homosexuals, however, coming out implies the risk of severing family ties, not so much because families would explicitly reject or disinherit them, but rather because there is a deeply ingrained feeling that being homosexual hurts the family, that is, causes shameful pain to those whom you love most. It is for this reason that many Latinos can come out to themselves and others only by moving far away from the family and keeping the "deep and dark" secret away from loved ones, in a hopeful, "out of sight, out of mind" fashion. At times, the paths of migration and exile are embraced as the only way out of this personal dilemma between family loyalty and same-sex desire. However, migration and exile constitute only a fragile, temporary cure, achieved via geographical mobility, for a deeply felt conflict of personal shame and family relations.

It seems obvious that an intervention directed at Latino self-identified homosexuals must take into account this central issue regarding family relations, and the dire consequences of living congruently within the domains of self-identity, public identification, and sexual practice within Latino communities. These central issues for self-identified homosexuals are the very important issues that get swept under the carpet when addressing homogeneously same-sex behavior among MSM.

In my opinion, the bottom line is that addressing self-identified gay Latinos as MSM is deeply insensitive, insulting, and ultimately conspires with the homophobic silence that creates so much disruption, suffering, and risky behavior in our lives. The label MSM itself witnesses without challenge the cultural forces that promote public silence and personal shame about same-sex desire and behavior. Not to mention that, for many of us, heterosexually identified MSM have been the perpetrators of sexual abuse during childhood and early adolescence. Because adopting a gay identity within Latino communities constitutes a courageous defiance of the oppressive homophobia and machismo of the culture, it should be honored and supported rather than overlooked in the name of an all-inclusive MSM construct.

Research has shown that, among MSM, problems in self-identification as gay or homosexual is predictive of AIDS risk behavior (Seibt and McAlister, 1993). Interventions to reduce risk behavior, therefore, should help with the struggles against shame and social isolation involved in the process of gay self-identification and coming out. In contrast, the label MSM focuses superficially on the surface behavior reinforcing the split between behavior and identity; from my perspective, this is equivalent to promoting risky behavior. In the same way that heterosexual men who have sex with other men deserve respect for their identity and behavioral choices, self-identified gay men must be recognized for their attempts at congruence between self-identification and sexual behavior. Interventions designed for MSM do a poor job in supporting the latter.

A "Deficit" Pedagogy

When I read AIDS prevention posters, ads, or other marketing and educational materials, with the now familiar messages, Use Condoms; Protect Yourself; Get Tested; Play Safe, and so on, I can't help but focus on the linguistic form of the messages. Linguistically, those messages are considered "imperatives," a grammatical form with the explicit function of giving commands and promoting compliance. I would like to argue that AIDS education and prevention efforts that are based on commands and implicit (or quite explicit) requests for compliance, found too often in programs and materials directed specifically at minority populations, do not promote, but rather undermine, the exercise of responsible self-regulation within the domain of sexual activity. Furthermore, I would like to argue that a pedagogy of "command/compliance" is most likely to occur when clients are perceived as "deficient," that is, ignorant, incompetent, not motivated, sexually driven, or generally not capable of self-direction.

As a developmental psychologist, I am well aware that imperatives or commands are the trademark of what is known as "authoritarian" parenting styles, styles of childrearing based on strong parental authority, power assertion, and requests for unquestioned compliance. Developmental researchers have consistently documented the negative effects of authoritarian parenting styles on children's self-regulatory abilities and perceptions of competence. For example, adolescents raised in authoritarian families, in contrast to those raised by more democratic or collaborative parents, show lower levels of social and cognitive competence, poorer academic achievement, and, interestingly, a higher incidence of drug use (Baumrind, 1985).

In microanalytic studies of parent-child and teacher-student verbal communication, interactions that are highly controlling, characterized by adult power assertions and requests for passive compliance, tend to promote hostile acting out and discourage self-regulatory functioning. On the other hand, teaching interactions characterized by questions rather than commands, collaboration rather than children's passive observation, and frequent adult attributions of children's competence have positive consequences on the development of autonomy and self-regulation. Within the domain of moral development, for example, parent-child interactions characterized by collaborative inductive inquiry, rather than adult power assertions—that is, families where children are engaged in reasoning collaboratively with parents rather than told rules and directives that must be unquestioningly followed—lead to more mature levels of moral reasoning and behavior (Hoffman, 1970).

Developmental studies clearly suggest that presenting messages, information, or guidelines for appropriate behavior in terms of commands and requests for passive compliance does not allow the intelligent, reasoned, and active participation of individuals that is necessary for self-regulated functioning. The most likely reason is that commands, unlike collaborative inquiry and reasoning, are simply and superficially "introjected" by individuals rather than truly "internalized" (see, for example, Deci and Ryan, 1985). Superficially introjected commands, that is, compliance with commands recognized as externally given rather than self-formulated, is a fragile system for guiding behavior adaptively and flexibly in the face of challenging circumstances. Adaptive self-directed functioning, on the other hand, involves the successful internalization of rules and guidelines for appropriate social and sexual behavior. True internalization is possible only through individuals' active participation, personal construction, and self-formulation of behavioral guidelines and intentions. Thus, the successful socialization of persons into creative, productive, and self-directed members of society involves not a simple transmission of information, and rules to be introjected in the imperative form, but rather a collaborative co-construction of guidelines and intentions in active participation with parents, teachers, or more expert members of the culture.

My basic argument for the purpose of this book is that we must critically examine the teaching styles or pedagogy underlying our AIDS prevention and education activities, especially when those activities are directed to minority populations and, in particular, Latino gay men. Are we allowing our clients, our target population, to participate collaboratively in the active construction of behavioral intentions, or are we simply stating, repeating, and reinforcing a simplistic set of "do's" and "don'ts," couched in the imperative form? Populations, students, or children who are perceived as "not capable" or somehow "deficient" by government, educators, or parents will be most likely treated with commands and authoritarian interactions. This is a clear central finding, and most likely a causative factor, regarding the problems of school failure and school dropout for many minority children in our schools. Research shows that teacher discourse directed at minority children contains more imperatives, fewer questions, and less invitations or opportunities for active participation than the discourse directed at white, economically advantaged students.

AIDS prevention programs that are based on the notion that Latino gay men are "deficient" in either knowledge, motivation, or skill to practice safe sex run the risk of adopting education strategies that are authoritarian, condescending, and, ultimately, counterproductive to the promotion of responsible self-direction and self-regulation in sexual practices. Perhaps the enormous amount of relapse to unsafe practices among gay men is due in part to the fact that many have been attempting to sustain safer sex practices over time with a fragile system of introjected rules like "use condoms" and "play safe" rather than well-reasoned and self-formulated guidelines for sexual activity that could be flexibly enacted for their own particular talents, weaknesses, situations, or changing circumstances.

To the best of my knowledge, most interventions directed to Latino gay men in this country, as well as to many other populations at risk (with a few notable exceptions), have not examined their pedagogy in terms of authoritarian control or their effects on clients' self-regulation. Rather, following traditional public health models, and in the name of

"saving lives," programs have acted too often like authoritarian families. While the issue of "cultural sensitivity" can be found in almost any
AIDS-prevention writing or program design, a meritorious accom-
plishment in itself, the same coverage and attention to a possible deficit
pedagogy has received scant attention (see Wallerstein and Bernstein,
1994, for a notable exception). Should we then be surprised by fragile
introjections, weak self-regulatory functioning, frequent relapses, defiance, and hostile acting out in safer sex practices? In Chapter 9, I will
offer my suggestions for less authoritarian and more empowering AIDS
education for Latino gay men.

"Risky" Sex as Natural and Meaningful Behavior

A major problem with many HIV risk-reduction interventions and
health education programs is their failure to acknowledge the profound
subjective meaning of unprotected sexual encounters. Four important
psychological dimensions of a sexual encounter—pleasure, connection,
affirmation, and exchange—are directly challenged by the introduction
of a latex barrier. The sense of pleasure and connection experienced by
contacting another human being's genitals, flesh-to-flesh, mucous
membrane-against-mucous membrane, with all the hardness, softness,
warmth, and wetness of sex, is definitely altered, if not seriously dis-
rupted, by the use of condoms. Because for many gay men a sexual
encounter provides an opportunity for affirming their attractiveness,
masculinity, and strength, the possibility of losing penile erection, due
to negative emotional and physical reactions to condoms, presents a
very real threat of substantial embarrassment: Condoms on flaccid
penises are not a beautiful sight! Moreover, the powerful and deeply
satisfying experience of semen exchange between two men, either
through oral ingestion or ejaculation inside the body, is definitely out of
the question with condom use under the threat of HIV transmission.
Thus, the latex barrier, though admittedly protective and life-saving, is
nonetheless *a barrier* for many important things other than HIV, and it
must be honestly treated at such. *Al pan pan y al vino vino* (literally,
"Call bread bread, and wine wine," a Spanish phrase conveying the
notion that things must be called by their true names—that is, truth
must be told even if difficult consequences must be faced).

A fascinating study of 64 Norwegian gay men by sociologist A. Prieur

(1990) vividly brings to our attention the disruptive impact of condoms on the sexual satisfaction involved in gay sex:

> As Olav observes: "What's the point with a condom? The whole point is that it [semen] should go inside you, otherwise you haven't given him all of yourself." When he sucks he insists that his partners come in his mouth: "If you don't swallow it, you haven't given him anything." . . . Accepting semen has been an important value in the gay culture, a way of showing devotion and belonging. . . . "The best thing that you could do for somebody was to swallow their semen. Now it's the opposite." (pp. 113–114)

As cited by Prieur (1990), the work of American anthropologist L. Kochems (1987) converges on the same findings:

> Informants have expressed to me that intercourse without a condom brings them "closer," it's more "intimate." They often express the desire for a "feeling of oneness" or "sharing." Expressions like "I want you inside me" or "I need you to cum in me," "I want to cum in you, to be part of you," as phrases used in sexual encounters indicate a desire for a joining, a oneness or incorporation in one another's physical being. (p. 8)

I have found similar voices among the Latino gay men I interviewed in San Francisco:

> *Cuando finalmente llegué a la meta final de deshacerme de todos los cachibaches morales, sociales y culturales y qué sé yo qué más . . . cuando llegué finalmente al punto de quitarme todo eso y llegué a la meta, me encontré que no puedo cobrar el premio porque existe esta situación del SIDA. Lo que él menciona de abandonarse en un momento sexual, eso describe bastante bien como yo me siento en una situación sexual. Realmente me enfurece la situación de tener que parar y decir bueno, "ok, condom time" . . . Cuando me encuentro en la situación [sexual] con mi compañero, soy un hombre que está haciendo el amor a otro hombre y no tengo que tener miedo de que alguien me va a hacer esto o a hacer lo otro. Es una mezcla de victoria, una situación bastante "empowering," es una sensación de eso es lo que soy y se siente tan bien y lo estoy haciendo conforme a lo que nace de mí, y hay una persona*

*conmigo que está compartiendo mis mismas emociones y compartiendo
lo que nos gusta y compartiendome y compartiendonos. Esto es algo
muy poderoso para mí. Y en un momento sexual la idea del semen es
todavía más poderosa para mí . . . lo único que puedo decir es que la
idea de tener una parte, una parte viviente, de esa persona dentro de
mí es muy poderosa. Recuerdo que cuando yo era un chico, la primera
vez que alguien eyaculó dentro de mí, yo era un jovencito recuerdo que
me causó una impresión muy fuerte, qué es esto? . . . observé placer en
la persona, y sentí, lo sentí dentro de mí. Desde ese punto empecé a
pensar: Está vivo y es una parte viviente dentro de mí, es él, una parte
de él dentro de mí . . . es una idea que "blows my mind" . . . es lo máx-
imo que no puedo pasar más allá. . . . Entonces cuando te encuentras
en una situación que ahora no puedes experimentar, alcanzar esa cima
en la intimidad con otra persona, realmente me encoleriza.*

(When I finally got to the finish line, and I was able to get rid of
all this baggage and inhibitions—moral, social, and cultural—I
realized that I can't get the prize because of AIDS. What he mentioned about abandoning yourself in a sexual situation describes
very well how I feel in a sexual situation. Really, what makes me
angry is to stop and have to say, "OK, condom time." When I am
in a sexual situation with my partner, I am a man that is making
love to another man, and I shouldn't have to be afraid that he's
going to give me this or that. It's a mixture of victory and
empowerment, it is the feeling that I am being who I am, I am
doing what I like, what feels spontaneous and natural for me, and
there is this person with me that is sharing my same emotions,
and sharing what we like, and sharing me, and sharing us. This is
something very powerful for me. And in the moment of sex, the
idea of semen is even more powerful for me . . . the only thing I
can say is that having a part, a living part, of that person inside
me is very powerful. I remember that when I was a child, the first
time that someone ejaculated inside me when I was a youngster, I
remember that it made a big impression on me, I said, what's
that? I observed pleasure in that other person, I felt him inside
me, and from that time on I thought, "He is alive, he is a living
part inside me" . . . it's an idea that blows my mind. . . . It's the
greatest thing, and I can't go beyond it. . . . Now when you find

yourself in the situation that now you can't experience, that you can't reach that peak in intimacy with another person, it really makes me mad.)

Qualitative observations by sociologists and anthropologists have been validated in quantitative research. For example, research psychologist J. Kelly et al., (1991) surveyed a convenience sample of 470 gay bar patrons in four U.S. cities. Of the men surveyed, a total of 209 (45% labeled "lapsers") reported at least one instance of unprotected intercourse during the six months prior to the survey. Lapsers were asked to rate the importance of 21 situations associated with their most recent instance of unprotected intercourse. The highest rating was given to the situational descriptor "This partner was someone special to me"; the second highest rating was given for the situation "I wanted to please my partner."

Thus, research findings across disciplines and across methodologies point to the serious disruption of closeness, satisfaction, and connection that condom use represents to many gay men in the U.S. and abroad. It is no surprise, therefore, that young gay men report higher rates of unprotected intercourse with their boyfriends or primary partners (Kegeles, Hays, and Coates, 1996), that prostitutes are less likely to use condoms with their lovers than with their clients (Day and Ward, 1990), and that a major problem in HIV prevention is presented by HIV serodiscordant couples, where non-infected partners continue to avoid protection in full knowledge and awareness of their risk of infection (Remien, Carballo-Diéguez, and Wagner, 1995).

This need for deeply felt interpersonal connection in a sexual encounter is more urgent for those men who feel a sense of social alienation and little social support, as is sadly the case of many Latino gay men I interviewed. These men are typically caught in social isolation between the homophobia of their families and native communities on one hand, and the racism of the mainstream gay community on the other. Often, isolated individuals who do not feel good about themselves may seek in sexual encounters a sense of social connection and personal validation that is subjectively experienced as more important than the use of a protective barrier. This is precisely what Prieur found in her studies: Those men with fewer sources of social support reported a greater need for connection through instances of unprotected intercourse.

In contrast, and understandably so, HIV educators have attempted to create a prevention culture where condoms are seen as fun, colorful, sexy; a culture where condom use is purposefully presented as the accepted "group norm"; a culture where negative feelings and attitudes toward condoms are not politically correct and better remain unsaid. Rarely do we see a frank recognition that condoms are not natural, that latex is artificial and doesn't quite feel good, at least at the beginning, and that indeed condoms are experienced by many as a barrier to flesh-to-flesh closeness and connection. To push condoms to our clients without recognition and validation of their subjective experience is to alienate and ignore the actual experience of many who have tried and struggled to incorporate condoms with difficulty into their sexual practices.

From the beginning, lacking in recognition and validation, the health educator messenger who pushes such simplistic messages about condoms is seen as dishonest, not to be trusted, as someone who is not interested in clients' feelings, experiences, struggles. It would be so much more honest to validate the negative feelings—the whole range of disappointing, embarrassing, unpleasurable sensations, and feelings of deprivation, both physical and psychological! Only once these are acknowledged and recognized, the questions can be posed: How can we make it feel better? What other ways can we experience the lost pleasurable sensation, the closeness, the connection, the bond? How can we befriend these inanimate latex creatures that, to date, are our only hope and protection from HIV infection? Only those whom we have truly listened to and whose experience we have validated will remain present to meet the challenges posed by these questions.

I must admit that as I was writing the above paragraphs, I was filled with ambivalence and doubt. By acknowledging and showing respect to the difficulties created by the latex barrier, am I encouraging unpro-tected sex? Am I discouraging condom use? My deepest conviction, however, is that we will not be able to collaborate with (so-called) lapsers in their adoption of safer sex intentions and practices until we meet them where they really are. After all, the cardinal rule of effective social work is "Begin where your client is." Attempts to silence their voices of frustration and disgust toward condoms will only result in fur-ther alienation of this group of men from badly needed education and prevention activities. A denial of gay men's negative feelings, and of the space to share them in all their brutal power, will only promote a further dissociation of sexual feelings from the intelligent, rational, self-regulatory guidance of behavior. In other words, contrary to the desired outcome of erotization and adoption of condoms, the denial and silence of negative attitudes toward condoms will only widen the gaps between HIV knowledge, intention, and behavior.

The incredible and admirable human capacity *gradually* to transform a barrier into a friendly, erotic, and welcome sexual toy can be achieved only by acknowledging first the condom's true nature as an annoying and disruptive barrier. I have italicized the word gradually to underscore the fact that the adoption and erotization of condoms is a process that takes time and effort. We need to collaborate respectfully with gay men's gradual erotization of condoms. We need to collaborate with their personal and active construction of safer sex intentions, and further collaborate with them in their struggles to enact those intentions. Respectful collaboration is not possible if we don't deeply listen to these men, and if these men don't feel deeply listened to. I am afraid that the needed erotization of condoms will not occur simply by pairing cute guys and condoms in a Pavlovian fashion, nor by the threat of sexual deprivation—No glove, No love—so prevalent in HIV prevention materials directed at gay men.

Signs of Spring

I am happy to report that in the last few years, and through the CDC funding of organizations such as the National Latino/a Lesbian and Gay Organization (LLEGO), the National Task Force on AIDS Prevention (NTFAP), and the Mission Neighborhood Health Center (MNHC) in San Francisco, and fueled by the initiatives and efforts of highly creative and committed Latino gay men, innovative programs have begun to emerge. In San Francisco, programs such as "Colegio contra SIDA" (a program of Proyecto contra SIDA por Vida), "El Ambiente" (a program of the Latino gay organization AGUILAS), and "Hermanos de Luna y Sol" (a program of the Mission Neighborhood Health Center) have been designed to address the social, interpersonal, and cultural contexts that promote risk behavior, taking into account the meaning of sexual practices from the unique perspective of Latino gay men. These programs promote the healthy integration of a dual minority identity, gay and Latino, within a supportive community of peers. Even though we do not have yet convincing evaluation data on these programs, these interventions do not suffer from the gaps described in the preceding paragraphs. In Chapter 9, I will discuss one of these programs, *Hermanos de Luna y Sol*, in some detail, as a model for AIDS education and prevention for our community.

Limitations of Current Research with Latino Gay Men

If readers are discouraged by the fact that most HIV prevention interventions for Latino gay men to date have been limited in serious ways, maybe they should skip the following section. The news about research on Latino gay men, research that could potentially guide and inform the design and implementation of future HIV risk-reduction interventions, is definitely worse.

In the summer of 1992, I was granted a two-year post-doctoral fellowship to study AIDS-prevention research at the Center for AIDS Prevention Studies, University of California San Francisco (CAPS/UCSF). I began my studies by examining the existing literature on Latino gay men. I was dumbfounded. Ten years into the AIDS epidemic, with full public awareness that HIV infection is running rampant among gay men of color, empirical studies of Latino gay men could be counted with the fingers of one hand. Moreover, of the four existing AIDS "knowledge-attitude-behavior" studies, only one of them attempted some kind of probabilistic/representative sampling strategy (NTFAP, 1993), and only one of them had been published—published only in Spanish, in the *Latin American Journal of Psychology* (Sabogal et al., 1992), not quite accessible to health educators, intervention designers, and policymakers responsible for HIV prevention in the U.S. As I will review with greater detail in Chapter 3, the situation has improved somewhat, though not enough, considering this high-risk and poorly understood population. In that first encounter with the research literature during the summer of 1992, it was painful to realize that there were many more studies of Latino heterosexuals than of Latino homosexuals, even though the latter carry the weight of the epidemic.

Fortunately, qualitative studies in the form of ethnographic studies and clinical reports appeared in higher, though still limited, numbers during my literature search. Of special value were the studies of anthropologist Joseph Carrier, whose detailed observations of homosexual and bisexual men in the U.S.-Mexican border represent an oasis of insight in a desert of ignorance. Above all, the qualitative work of Joe Carrier, Raúl Magaña, Eduardo Morales, Tomás Almaguer, and other pioneers in the field have alerted readers that Latino homosexuals are very different from Euro-American gay men on a wide range of variables relevant to HIV prevention, such as the meaning of what constitutes homosexual behavior, the degree of identification with the gay community, the sources of social support, and the processes involved in dual-minority identity formation as both Latinos and gay men in the U.S. But, unfortunately, qualitative and quantitative research on Latino gay men have remained on parallel tracks with little interaction or cross-fertilization.

Quantitative research, shaped mostly by academic models of health risk and behavior change, rather than by culturally grounded models of sexual "risky" behavior, has typically investigated the same questions asked of mainstream (mostly White) gay men. The voices of Latino gay and bisexual men, their subjective experiences and struggles in the AIDS epidemic, as well as the sociocultural cultural forces that shape them, have remained painfully absent in the lean body of quantitative research. One notable exception is the recently published work of Alex Carballo-Diéguez, to be reviewed with detail in Chapter 2.

The picture gets even grimmer if we look at the published literature in search of HIV risk-reduction intervention research. By intervention research I mean literature that reports the design, implementation, and outcome evaluation of HIV risk-reduction strategies targeted to this population, with the use of reliable measures of behavior change and in the context of research designs with documented experimental validity. Well, there are none! I think this is a scandal that should provoke rage among Latino gay men, especially in light of the fact that there are already a significant number of tested interventions targeting White gay men, African American adolescents, and Latino heterosexuals.

In chapters 1 and 2, I will review with greater detail the existing literature, both quantitative and qualitative, regarding HIV risk in Latino gay men. For now, the main point I want to underscore can be stated as follows: Effective HIV risk-reduction interventions must address the variables that promote and foster high-risk behavior. In other words, and in research parlance, interventions must address variables that "predict" safer or unsafe sexual behavior. To date, only three published studies have examined and tested predictors of risk among Latino gay men. In light of such limited information on predictors of risk, and zero information on scientifically tested interventions, we can conclude that thus far the research enterprise has failed Latino gay and bisexual men in their struggles with the AIDS epidemic.

The Purpose and Organization of the Present Book

After seriously criticizing both interventions and research, what do I or this book have to offer? I believe I can offer a fourfold contribution. First, I present a thorough and critical review of the existing literature. Second, I develop a cultural model of HIV risk, based on the voices and subjective experiences of Latino gay men as they struggle to practice safer sex in difficult situations. Third, I formalize the findings into a "psycho-cultural" model of sexual self-regulation; the model integrates the facts that sexuality is both culturally regulated and self-regulated. Finally, I share the experience of an HIV-prevention intervention, targeted to Latino gay men, that addresses the cultural barriers to safer sex and promotes sexual self-regulation in a culturally sensitive fashion.

The overall goal of the book is to provide a framework for HIV prevention in Latino gay and bisexual men from the point of view of a Latino gay man who is also a developmental psychologist, a behavioral researcher, and a social activist for all gay men of color. The book's overall hypothesis is that six sociocultural factors in the lives of Latino gay men—machismo, homophobia, family loyalty, sexual silence, poverty, and racism—internalized through socialization experiences, undermine the self-regulation of sexuality and have become important barriers to the practice of safer sex. Thus, I propose that "unsafe" sex does not simply reflect a deficit of knowledge, motivation, or skills in Latino gay men but rather that it is sexual behavior that has logic and meaning from a given sociocultural perspective.

The book is organized as follows. First, I present a review of the epidemiological (Chapter 1) and behavioral (Chapter 2) research to date, as it relates to HIV in Latino gay men (or MSM, when reviewing government-collected statistics). Following the review, I discuss in detail the fluid relation between safer sex intentions and actual safer sex behavior, with special attention to specific cultural factors that undermine the enactment of safer sex intentions (Chapter 3). In Chapters 4,

5, and 6 I bring the developmental histories, subjective experiences and voices of Latino gay men to the forefront of the discussion. These three chapters are organized around the six sociocultural factors that shape, regulate, and give meaning to sexual practices in our community. Chapter 7 offers a brief and limited discussion of variability within the population due to different degrees of acculturation to the mainstream, English-speaking community. In Chapter 8, I present the theoretical psycho-cultural model of sexual self-regulation that integrates the tension between cultural regulation and self-regulation of sexuality. And finally, in Chapter 9, I provide an example of how the sociocultural model can guide an effective HIV prevention intervention with this population.

The review chapters (1 and 2) are heavy with quantitative data and discuss with detail issues of measurement and methodological concerns typical of survey research. For those readers who are turned off by language labeled by some as "researcherese," or who simply are not interested in figures, statistics, or methodological details, I suggest skipping these two chapters and reading only the summary of quantitative findings given at the end of Chapter 2 (p. 47). If skipped, the review chapters could also be used as future reference for specific statistics, percentages, and rates for different variables, under each of the appropriate headings that might be of interest to different readers. In my opinion, the "soul" of the book is found in Chapters 4 through 7; these chapters are the closest to the voices of the target community, while a specific path toward creative prevention efforts is given in Chapter 9.

It is my hope that the ideas presented in this book will not only guide future innovative and effective interventions to reduce the spread of AIDS in our community, but also inspire and guide further behavioral research. In the ideal world, the main assumptions and hypotheses of the theoretical framework proposed in this book would be further tested for their validity in predicting HIV risk behavior and for their generalizability across the different segments and subgroups that comprise the diverse population of Latino gay and bisexual men in the U.S. I am happy to report that the Office of AIDS Research (OAR) and the National Institute of Child Health and Human Development (NICHD) of the National Institutes of Health (NIH) have recently funded a research program to develop and empirically test the main assumptions and hypotheses proposed in this book. The funding will support a qualitative study, a quantitative survey, and the development of an intervention based on the data collected. I will be devoting the next four years of my research to this important endeavor. Needless to say, I welcome from other researchers and practitioners such questioning, testing, and application of any or all of the propositions advanced in this book.

The Nature of My Evidence

The observations, quotes, theoretical statements, and hypotheses presented in this book emerge from an integration of data from five different sources:

1. A thorough and critical review of the published epidemiological and behavioral science literature that have presented, both quantitatively and qualitatively, empirical data on Latino gay men;
2. A qualitative study focused on sexuality and HIV transmission, conducted in San Francisco during the 1992–1993 academic year, when I interviewed approximately 70 Latino self-identified gay and bisexual men in the context of focus groups and individual in-depth interview;
3. A quantitative survey with Latino gay men in Tucson (n=159) done in collaboration with researchers at the Center of AIDS Prevention Studies (CAPS), and a survey of Latino gay men in San Francisco (n=109) done in collaboration with Dr. Eduardo Morales from the California School of Professional Psychology;
4. In-depth interviews conducted in early 1996 with 32 self-identified Latino gay men, as part of San Francisco's "Qualitative Interview Study" (QIS), sponsored by the San Francisco AIDS Foundation and conducted in collaboration with researchers at CAPS. Among other things, the QIS study elicited from participants detailed narratives of sexual episodes of both protected and unprotected anal intercourse; and
5. Last but not least, my own personal participation and involvement with the Latino gay community and with community-based organization serving this population, at both national and local levels. I have participated and continue to participate in the community as a member, as a researcher focused on HIV prevention research with

Latino gay men, and as a consultant, collaborator, and/or group facilitator in several community-based HIV prevention programs. I have attended conferences and activities of the National Latino/a Lesbian and Gay Organization (LLEGO), especially sessions, workshops, and special meetings devoted to HIV prevention in the community, as well as attended several annual institutes on Gay Men of Color and AIDS sponsored by the National Task Force on HIV Prevention (NTFAP). I have learned the most precious lessons through this participant observation, and the book, as well as my researcher perspective, has been greatly enriched by this participation and close observation of the struggles of this community with a devastating epidemic.

I must also confess that this book reflects my own personal experience as a Latino gay man whose life and sexuality has been impacted by the sociocultural factors presented in this book as well as by the AIDS epidemic. I speak about someone who, although HIV-negative to date, has been deeply affected by multiple losses and a great deal of suffering due to AIDS. I speak first-hand as someone who has had to struggle with the practice of safer sex and whose attempts at protection have failed many times. My serious concerns about objectivity and my desire to speak above all about my community rather than just about myself must be tempered with the fact that ". . . all attempts at theorizing social life are, at the same time, works of autobiography" (Simon, 1996, p.1).

A Note on the Target Population

For very important reasons, most sections of this book purposefully refer to *Latino gay men*, or to *Latino gay and bisexual men* rather than to Latino *men who have sex with men* (MSM).

First, in most of the studies to be reviewed in Chapters 1, 2, and 3, the majority of respondents have self-identified as gay, homosexual, or bisexual. Thus, the findings refer to groups of Latino men who, for the most part, experience some connection or congruence between their sexual behavior and their sexual identity. It should be clear, however, that many of these *self*-identified respondents are not necessarily *publicly* identified, and we must remember that many in our community still remain or are forced to remain in the homophobic closet with respect to family, co-workers, and even friends.

A second reason is that, for self-identified gay men, the meaning, context, and subjective experience of same-sex behavior are qualitatively different than for those MSM who do not identify as such. For example, when study participants report that condoms do not "feel" the same, readers should be aware that, in self-identified gay men, many of these "feelings" refer not only to pleasurable sensations but also more importantly to a deep desire for close, deeply felt, affectionate, and romantic encounters between gay and bisexual men that a latex barrier is perceived to disturb.

As I discussed earlier in the chapter, we know that in Latino communities, as well as in many other communities, there are men whose same-sex behavior has no impact on their heterosexual identity. And it is for this reason, and due to the fact that HIV is transmitted through behaviors and not identities, that the label MSM is widely, and sometimes appropriately, used. However, the fact remains that the overwhelming majority of participants in the studies reviewed below *do* self-identify as gay or bisexual, and the findings do not apply to the more generic, over-inclusive, MSM category. Heterosexually identified MSM must be studied on their own terms. I will use the label MSM only when it is specifically needed, as when reporting government-collected statistics on AIDS cases and HIV seroprevalence in Chapter 1.

In addition, for reasons of convenience and style, I have taken the liberty of using the word gay in its most inclusive form, namely, to refer to men who have sex with other men and who also identify personally and publicly as other than heterosexual. Thus, in this book, the term *Latino gay men* refers to men who may identify themselves as homosexual, bisexual, transgender, queen, *buchona, joto, pato, maricón*, or any other of the multiple ways in which Latino men attempt to find congruence between their sexual behavior and their sexual identity. The majority of these men would agree that they are not heterosexual and that they are part of a gay world or live a gay life. Even though my analyses have attempted to focus on the commonality of experiences within an extremely diverse group of men, my use of the word gay should *not* be taken to indicate that such diversity, coded in the colorful labels of identities and self-definitions, is less relevant or unimportant. I must admit, however, that this book is more about commonality than diversity.

1.

Findings
of Epidemiological
Research

Based on epidemiological studies of HIV, I would like to assess the degree of risk that Latino gay men in the U.S. experience with respect to HIV transmission. Whenever possible, the assessment will be done in comparison to groups of non-Latino gay and bisexual men. First, I will review both the absolute numbers and the rates of increase of diagnosed AIDS cases among Latino men who have sex with men, as reported by the CDC and other government health agencies. Second, I will review the current estimates of HIV infection in our community, as determined by studies of HIV seroprevalence (i.e., studies that involved testing of blood samples). Finally, I will review self-reported rates of sexual risk behavior, such as unprotected anal intercourse, that continue to threaten many members of this community with new infections.

The statistics that follow will give us a clear and unequivocal indication that our community of Latino gay men, in comparison to other communities in the U.S., has been *severely* affected by the AIDS epidemic. The numbers tell us that for many years we have been, and remain, a group at an extremely high risk for the transmission of HIV.

AIDS Cases among Latino Men Who Have Sex with Men

As overlapping members of two high-risk groups (Latinos and men who have sex with men), Latino gay men in the U.S. have been highly and disproportionately affected by the AIDS epidemic. During 1990, death rates (per 100,000) for HIV-related causes was 22.2 for Latinos compared to 8.7 for Whites (NCA, 1992). By June 1996, 18% of all diagnosed AIDS cases in the country were Latino, an ethnic group that constitutes only about 9% of the U.S. population (CDC, 1996). Similarly, since the beginning of the HIV epidemic, men who have sex with men have carried the largest and most disproportionate share of AIDS cases in the nation; as of June 1996, 67% of all male diagnosed AIDS cases in the U.S. have been among MSM.

Also as of June 1996, a total of 40,243 AIDS cases have been diagnosed among Hispanic/Latino men who have sex with men; Latino MSM thus constitute 51% of all reported Latino male AIDS cases in the nation (CDC, 1996). Percentages of Latino AIDS cases accounted for by MSM vary substantially across the three major ethnic subgroups. In 1992, for example, 70% of Cuban, 59% of Mexican, and 18% of Puerto Rican AIDS cases were among MSM (CDC, 1993a). The relatively low percentage of MSM among Puerto Rican AIDS cases reflects the higher incidence of HIV transmission through injection drug use in this population. Many of the Puerto Rican drug-related cases, however, could also be MSM, though not coded as such by the CDC.

The number of diagnosed AIDS cases in the nation continues to increase at a faster and disproportionate rate among Latino than non-Latino White men who have sex with men. For example, by March 1993, a total of 21,021 AIDS cases had been diagnosed in Latino MSM (CDC, 1993b); by June 1994, 15 months later, the number of diagnosed Latino MSM AIDS cases had risen to 29,432. Thus, in the 15 months between March 1993 and June 1994, AIDS diagnosed cases increased about 40% among Latino gay and bisexual men (CDC, 1994). This large percentage increase should be examined in comparison to a much slower, though also painfully dramatic, 29% increase of AIDS cases in non-Latino White MSM during the same time period. The most recent statistics show that, in the two year period between July 1994 and June 1996, the number of diagnosed AIDS cases among Latino gay and bisexual men in the U.S. increased by 37%.

The numbers are even more striking when one examines those for cities with a high concentration of Latinos and homosexuals. In San Francisco, for example, the number of Latino AIDS cases diagnosed annually increased from 168 cases in 1989 to 334 in 1992; approximately 80% of these cases were Latino gay and bisexual men. These numbers are the lowest estimates possible because they are from the period before the CDC's major change in the diagnostic definition of AIDS, and are not corrected to include the broader, more inclusive current definition. The dramatic increase in AIDS cases among Latino gay and bisexual men stands in contrast to the slower, though also unfortunate, increase of cases for non-Latino Whites in the city during the same time period (an increase from 1,533 cases in 1989 to 2,239 in 1992; of these cases, 87% are gay and bisexual males). In other words, the number of yearly reported AIDS cases in the city increased 99% for Latinos but only 46% for non-Latino Whites within the same four-year period.

It should be noted that the statistics for Latino gay and bisexual men presented throughout this section are most likely conservative estimates for two important reasons. First, Lindan et al. (1990) have shown that, in California, about 20% of Latino AIDS cases were incorrectly reported and recorded as non-Latino Whites. Second, as recently recognized by the National Commission on AIDS (NCA, 1992), different definitions of homosexuality and gay identity among Latinos "may skew statistics dealing with homosexual/bisexual infection rates since there are Hispanic/Latino men who fit these categories but do not identify themselves accordingly" (p. 40).

HIV Prevalence and Seroconversion

While the epidemiological trends are somewhat clear for diagnosed AIDS cases, there are no reliable epidemiological studies of HIV seroprevalence, seroconversion, or both among Latino gay and bisexual men that involve probabilistic, representative samples. *Seroprevalence* refers to estimates of how many persons are HIV positive in a given population, while *seroconversion* refers to the proportion of men from the population who become HIV positive ("convert") during a given time period. Seroprevalence and seroconversion studies estimate the prevalence and incidence respectively, of HIV based on analysis of blood samples rather than on participants' self-report.

Data from two seroprevalence studies in the U.S. clearly show that Latinos (regardless of risk category or sexual orientation) are more likely to be infected with HIV than are non-Latino Whites. One study, done with economically disadvantaged Job Corps entrants, revealed that Latinos were infected at a rate two and a half times higher than Whites (St. Louis et al., 1991). In a second study, done with active-duty members of the U.S. army, Latinos were three times more likely than non-Latino Whites to be HIV infected (Kelley et al., 1990). Even though these two seroprevalence studies did not distinguish gay and bisexual from other types of cases, the data are consistent with the findings that Latino gay and bisexual men are highly and disproportionately affected by the HIV epidemic.

Most of what we know about HIV seroprevalence and seroconversion, specifically among Latino gay men, comes from studies of (mostly) White gay men that have included relatively small numbers of Latinos. One important longitudinal study of seroconversion among gay men (Kingsley, 1991) is indicative of both the seriousness of the problem and the limitations of our current data on Latino gay men. The Multicenter AIDS Cohort Study (MACS) followed the temporal trends in HIV seroconversion among gay males in five major urban centers in the U.S. between 1984 and 1989. The study included a total of 3,262 originally HIV-negative gay men, of whom approximately 90 were Latino. Overall, when compared to White gay men, Latino gay men showed a higher HIV seroconversion rate in the city of Los Angeles and a much higher rate—330% higher!—in the city of Chicago. However, the small proportion (2.7%) of Latinos in the study, the English-only questionnaires, and the fact that Hispanic Blacks were categorized as African Americans make the findings difficult to interpret. If at all valid, the reported rates for Latinos are most likely conservative estimates of true seroconversion rates in our communities. Nevertheless, because epidemiological studies of seroconversion rates are difficult and expensive to do, the present data constitute highly prized information on the largely unknown and understudied population of Latino gay males.

Based on numerous epidemiological studies in the region, the AIDS Office of the San Francisco Department of Health has estimated the HIV seroprevalence among Latino gay and bisexual men in San Francisco at 43% (SFDH, 1993); that is, *close to one-half* of Latino gay and bisexual men in San Francisco are infected with HIV! Seroprevalence for non-Latino White gay and bisexual men in the city is slightly lower, estimated at 41%. Considering that the HIV epidemic first started and rapidly spread in San Francisco's White gay community, a seroprevalence of 43% among Latino gay and bisexual men indicates not only that HIV infection has caught up with the Latino gay and bisexual community but also that it is increasing at a faster rate in this population. This observation is confirmed by a 1992 seroprevalence study of *young* gay and bisexual men, ages 18 to 29, in San Francisco, involving a multistage probability sample. The study showed a seroprevalence rate of 25% among the Latino young men, in contrast to a rate of 15.5% among the White young men (Osmond, Page, Wiley, et al., 1994).

Rates of Unprotected Intercourse

For clearly established biological reasons, and as confirmed by clear epidemiological findings, anal intercourse without condoms (i.e., unprotected anal intercourse) is recognized as one of the most efficient routes for the transmission of HIV. Unfortunately, studies done to date converge on the finding that Latino gay and bisexual men have had enormous difficulties adjusting to condom use and adopting less risky forms of sexual behavior. In fact, five studies that have measured rates of unprotected anal intercourse in gay and bisexual men (Doll et al., 1991; Fairbank, Bregman, and Maullin, 1991; Lemp, 1994; NTFAP, 1993; Richwald et al., 1988) show that Latinos had the highest rates of unprotected anal intercourse when compared to samples of non-Latino Whites, African Americans, or men from other minority groups.

For example, in a survey of knowledge, attitudes, and behavior conducted in the summer of 1990 in San Francisco's American Indian, Filipino, and Latino gay and bisexual male communities, Latinos reported the highest rate of unprotected anal intercourse (35%) during the last thirty days as compared to 25% of Filipinos and 12% of American Indians (Fairbank, Bregman, and Maullin, 1991). This situation has not changed much for Latinos in San Francisco during the last few years, even though AIDS education and prevention programs in the city are well established and are often regarded as state-of-the-art programs. In Lemp and associates' (1993) recent study of young gay men in San Francisco, 40% of Latinos reported engaging in unprotected anal intercourse during the last six months, as compared to 38% of African Americans and 28% of non-Latino Whites.

A similar situation has been found in Southern urban cities, not considered AIDS epicenters, as evidenced in a recent study of gay men of color sponsored by the National Task Force on AIDS Prevention (NTFAP, 1993). Sampled in eight urban centers, in five different states ranging from Texas to Florida, Latinos reported the highest rates of both insertive and receptive anal intercourse without condoms. For insertive anal intercourse, 38% of Latinos reported engaging in this activity without condoms during the previous month, as compared to 32% of African Americans and 29% of non-Latino Whites. Differences were even more striking for receptive anal intercourse: 37% of Latinos, 21% of African Americans, and 25% of non-Latino Whites reported engaging in this activity without condoms during the previous month.

Studies of special groups, such as bathhouse patrons or STD patients, have replicated the findings regarding the HIV vulnerability of Latino gay and bisexual men. In a relatively early study of patrons exiting gay bathhouses in Los Angeles, Richwald et al. (1988) found that, of all ethnic groups interviewed, Latinos accounted for the greatest proportion of men practicing anal sex without condoms. Approximately 25% (20/81) of Latinos interviewed reported engaging in unprotected anal intercourse during the bathhouse visit, as compared to 10% (10/99) of African American, and 9% (50/576) of White men. Finally, when predicting anal sex without condoms in predominantly Hispanic and Black clients of urban STD clinics, Doll et al. (1991) found three major predictors: number of drugs each month, sex within a steady relationship, and being of Latino/Hispanic ethnicity.

In the three most recent studies of Latino gay and bisexual men (Carballo-Diéguez, 1995a; Díaz et al., 1996; Ramírez, Suarez, de la Rosa, Castro, and Zimmerman, 1994), participants have reported extremely high rates of unprotected intercourse. Ramírez et al. (1994) surveyed 200 Mexican men in the border Mexican town of Juarez; because these men reported frequent contact with the gay community in the nearby U.S. town of El Paso, the data are informative about Latino gay and bisexual behavior in the U.S. Ramírez inquired about condom use in two different ways: (a) the number of times that condoms were used in the last 10 sexual encounters, and (b) the frequency of condom use in anal intercourse and oral sex rated on a three-point scale of "never," "occasionally," or "frequently." For the whole sample, the mean number of times they used condoms in the last 10 encounters was 6.47.

For insertive anal intercourse, 45% reported condom use as "frequent," 30% as "occasional," and 25% as "never." For receptive anal intercourse, 46% reported condom us as "frequent," 27% as "occasional" and 27% as "never." These data suggest that more than 50% of Mexican gay and bisexual men who are sexually active in border U.S. towns, and who have a relatively high knowledge about HIV and AIDS, continue to practice both receptive and insertive anal intercourse without condoms.

In a study of mostly gay and bisexual Puerto Rican men in New York City, Carballo-Diéguez (1995) examined the rates of unprotected insertive and receptive anal intercourse by different partner types within a 12-month period. For insertive anal sex, 37% reported unprotected intercourse with lovers, 32% reported unprotected intercourse with one night stands, and 22% reported unprotected intercourse with other types of partners. For receptive anal sex, 34% had unprotected intercourse with lovers, 22% with one night stands, and 18% with other partner types.

In a recent study of 159 Latino gay men recruited from gay bars in Tucson, Arizona, Díaz et al. (1996) surveyed participants' sexual practices with both monogamous and non-monogamous partners during the previous 30 days and during the past year. Questionnaires were available only in English; this Latino sample is likely to over-represent highly acculturated, English-speaking men. The results showed that, during the previous 30 days, 22% of the sample engaged in unprotected intercourse with non-monogamous partners. In addition, 51% of the men reported at least one instance of unprotected anal intercourse during the previous year.

Díaz et al. (1996) also estimated the frequency of unprotected intercourse in the sample by examining the proportion of condom use only among those men who reported *any* anal intercourse during the last 30 days. For the month prior to testing, 61 men (or 38%) of the sample reported engaging in anal intercourse with their primary partners, and 45 men (or 28%) reported engaging in anal intercourse with casual (non-primary) partners. Taking these numbers as the base denominator, the reported proportion of *unprotected* anal intercourse in the sample was alarmingly high: 67% (41/61) of the men who reported anal intercourse with primary partners were unprotected, and 44% (20/45) who reported anal intercourse with casual partners were unprotected during the previous 30 days.

Research findings in Tucson suggest that the majority of Latinos who are being safe are perhaps remaining so by abstaining, at least temporarily, from anal intercourse. However, when the men engage in anal intercourse, especially with primary partners, they typically have unprotected sex. The main concern with this strategy is that safety through abstinence might be a fragile way to maintain safer sex behavior over time. It is possible that abstinence from anal sex might mask a deeper aversion and inability to use condoms in an effective yet pleasurable manner.

An important finding in Díaz et al. (1996) study was that HIV risk behavior correlated negatively with both education and income, that is, within this sample there was more risky behavior in men that had less education and income. Because the men sampled were highly acculturated, English-speaking, and mostly well-educated, we should then expect higher rates of unprotected intercourse in less acculturated, Spanish-speaking men of lower socioeconomic status and lower education. This concern is based not only on the correlations between socioeconomic variables and risk behavior obtained in the Tucson study, but also on the documented relationship between acculturation and positive attitudes toward condom use among Latino heterosexuals (Marín, Tschann, and Gómez, 1993). Unfortunately, there are at present no systematic studies on the relationships among poverty status, education, acculturation, and HIV risk behavior among Latino gay and bisexual men.

In summary, studies have shown that Latino gay and bisexual men engage in extremely high rates of unprotected intercourse; that is, within a one-year period, about one-half of Latino gay and bisexual men in the U.S. engage in behavior that puts them at risk for HIV infection. The rates of men who practice risky sexual behavior vary, according to the window of time observed, from 23% to 35% (within one month) to about 40% (within six months) and about 50% (within a year). Although the largest proportion of unsafe sex appears to occur within steady-partner relationships, the data also show that the majority (about two-thirds) of those relationships are non-monogamous (Díaz, Morales, Dilán, and Rodríguez, 1997) and that there are also substantial amounts of risky sex with casual partners. These high rates of unprotected anal intercourse are possibly due to difficulties with or negative reactions to condom use, rather than lack of knowledge or lack of desire, intentions, or both to protect oneself and others against HIV infection.

The literature just reviewed has raised three important concerns. First, the data suggest that there is in our community a deep aversion toward the use of condoms, to the point that many Latino gay men are using abstinence from anal intercourse as a preferred strategy for safety. The concern is that this abstinence strategy, simply masking the deeper aversion toward condoms, might be a successful solution only in the short term, and a fragile one to maintain over time. Second, the large number of steady relationships that are in fact non-monogamous not only might create a false illusion of safety but also could become an obstacle to a frank and open discussion and communication about sexuality with our sexual partners. Without this frank and open communication, we will not be able to collaborate with one another in our continued attempts toward increasingly safer sexual activities. Finally, there is a strong possibility that rates of risky behavior are much higher in Spanish-speaking men of lower socioeconomic status. Because there are virtually no data on Spanish-speaking gay and bisexual men who are less acculturated, among them many recent immigrants, our prevention strategies with this population might be extremely inadequate, failing to target the (as yet) unknown factors that put these men at risk.

2.

Findings of Behavioral Research

A major task of behavioral researchers in the HIV epidemic is to under-stand and explain why there is so much difficulty in the adoption of safer sex practices among groups at risk. For the most part, behavioral research in this area has been guided by models of behavior change, that is, psychological theories that specify necessary steps or processes in the adoption of new behavior in order to avoid health risks, such as the adoption of condoms to avoid HIV infection. A good summary of theories of behavior change that have guided HIV prevention research and practice to date can be found in Leviton (1989). Even though I will offer a substantive critique of current models of behavior change in the next chapter, it is important now to review the research findings from studies that, for the most part, have been guided by those models.

With respect to HIV prevention, a number of theories converge on the hypothesis that four steps are necessary to change risky sexual behavior or adopt safer sex practices (see e.g., Catania et al., 1990). First, people must have accurate *knowledge* about modes of HIV preven-tion and means of prevention. Second, such knowledge must be person-alized by a sense of *perceived risk*, that is, the accurate self-perception that one is vulnerable or at risk of HIV infection when practicing the risky behavior. Third, in light of correct knowledge and accurate per-ceptions of risk, people must formulate relatively strong *intentions* to perform safer sex and avoid risky behavior. Finally, safer sex intentions must be successfully *enacted*, or put into practice, in the face of difficult situations or competing circumstances such as peer pressure or the threat of losing sexual arousal (erections) with condom use.

Because a major aim of this review is to understand why there is so much difficulty with condom use among Latino gay men, it is essential that we review current knowledge about the four different stages of behavior change in our target population. Taking the point of view of psychological theories of behavior change, it is important to search for possible gaps in knowledge, perceived risk, intentions, and their enactment that might signal potential breakdowns in the steps toward the adoption of safer sex.

Knowledge

The most consistent finding in the available literature about Latino gay men is that risky behavior continues to occur in the presence of substantial knowledge about modes of HIV transmission and means of prevention.

Research findings indicating substantial, though not perfect, HIV and AIDS knowledge have been reported by Sabogal et al., (1991) in a study of 100 Latino gay men in San Francisco; by Amaro and Gornermann (1992) in a sample of 284 Latino self-identified gay men in the northeastern U.S. and Puerto Rico; by Ramírez et al. (1994) in a sample of 200 Mexican gay and bisexual men in the U.S.-Mexican border town of Juarez; and by the National Task Force on AIDS Prevention in a study of gay men, of whom 137 are Latino, in eight urban centers in the U.S.

Sabogal et al. (1991) reported that 89% of the sample agreed with the statement, "Condoms are the best protection for HIV." Moreover, when asked the question, "How much would you say you know about AIDS?" 70% of the men in the sample responded, "A great deal." Amaro and Gornermann (1992) reported that response rates for HIV knowledge items ranged between 75% and 98% correct, except for an item on saliva/kissing and sharing toothbrushes (58% correct). Ramírez and his collaborators (1994) reported a mean of 79% correct in the sample's response to four open-ended questions that assessed HIV and AIDS knowledge: (a) What is AIDS? (b) How is HIV (or AIDS) transmitted? (c) What are the symptoms of a person with AIDS? and (d) Do you know any test to detect HIV?

In the study of 137 Latino gay and bisexual men in eight southern cities conducted by the National Task Force on AIDS Prevention (NTFAP, 1993), participants were questioned about specific and detailed facts regarding safer sex and condom use. The men responded quite accurately to items assessing the effectiveness of latex versus lambskin condoms (78% correct) and the protection utility of non-oxynol-9 (83% correct). They were also mostly accurate in identifying that unprotected intercourse with withdrawal before ejaculation does not prevent transmission (82% correct), that the inserter top partner in unprotected intercourse is also at risk (83% correct), and that it is not possible to tell by appearances alone whether a sex partner has AIDS or not (85% correct).

Even though the findings regarding a relatively high level of AIDS knowledge are consistent across different studies, the available evidence has also uncovered some significant sources of confusion and misconceptions that should be taken into account for further study. For example, in both the San Francisco and southern states studies, Latino gay men expressed the belief that HIV can be transmitted by donating blood. Only 32% of the San Francisco sample and 56% of the southern sample of Latino gay men knew that HIV cannot be transmitted by giving blood.

Three other findings regarding AIDS knowledge and beliefs are of some serious concern. First, a large number of Latinos believe that the transmission of AIDS can be prevented by having only one partner; in the San Francisco study, 89% of the sample endorsed the statement that "not being promiscuous/having only one partner is the best protection from HIV" (as reported in a presentation by Sabogal et al., 1991). Even though multiple sex partners do indeed increase the likelihood of HIV infection, it does not necessarily follow that having one partner constitutes effective protection, especially in communities like San Francisco, where there is a relatively high prevalence of HIV. The belief that protection can be achieved simply by reducing the number of partners to one may promote unprotected practices within primary relationships that are in fact not monogamous and, therefore, constitute a potential risk with respect to HIV transmission.

A second finding that raises some concern is that, according to findings from the southern states survey, Latino gay men seem to believe that people are "likely to get AIDS from practicing sex, even if they use condoms the right way all the time." When posed as a true or false statement, only 36.3% of Latino men responded to it as "false"; 32.5% responded to it as "true" and 31.2% as "don't know," indicating a high degree of uncertainty (actually a random distribution of responses) regarding the protective value of condoms. Such belief, which could ultimately undermine consistent condom use, might be related to the strong messages of the Catholic church, among others, that abstinence is the only safe alternative.

It is quite possible that the belief that even protected sex might be dangerous for HIV transmission may indicate more accurate knowledge and concern about the possibility of condom failure. Latinos may indeed experience more condom failure because of lack of sophisticated knowledge about proper usage, lack of awareness about condoms' limited life span, and ignorance about the dangers posed by oil-based lubricants. For example, in the southern states survey, 30.7% of Latino gay men believed erroneously that "it is good to use Vaseline/oil to stop a condom from breaking during sex."

In summary, even though the available literature converges on the fact that Latino gay and bisexual men have a substantial amount of HIV and AIDS knowledge, and specific knowledge about condom use, the knowledge is not perfect. We must recognize that, on many knowledge questions that are extremely relevant to HIV prevention, Latino gay and bisexual men have scored on the average between C+ and B–, to use a familiar scale. The bottom line is that, on some important items of HIV and AIDS information, Latino gay and bisexual men have mediocre knowledge, confusion, or both; a substantial number of them are simply lacking in such information. There is no reason why our knowledge on these life-and-death concerns should be less than A+.

In addition, because the available studies are so few and involve non-representative samples for the most part, we do not know how knowledge is actually presented or distributed across the entire population of Latino gay men in the U.S. It is possible that knowledge is less available to men who do not actively participate in the gay community (such as younger men), less acculturated recent immigrants, and men who are in the homophobic closet; these men are typically less in contact with sources of information targeted appropriately to gay and bisexual men.

The main point of concern here is that, even though there is evidence of substantial knowledge on many aspects of transmission and prevention of HIV, we cannot stop at this time the necessary and continuing task of educating and informing different members of the Latino gay and bisexual community. We must continue educating our community regarding specific, detailed, and practical information about effective condom use. This is especially urgent for those who could be more isolated and those who are in the process of coming out, such as younger men or those threatened by the intense homophobia found in the Latino communities.

Perceived Risk

Two studies of Latino gay and bisexual men, one study in five U.S. southern states (NTFAP, 1993), and a recent study in San Francisco (Díaz et al., in preparation), have measured participants' perceived vulnerability or perceived personal risk to HIV infection. Fortunately, because the more recent San Francisco study used virtually the same four questions used by the southern states study, we are able to compare data across these two different samples. The 109 men in the San Francisco sample live in an AIDS "epicenter"; these men, therefore, have been exposed to a great deal of information and mass media campaigns about HIV prevention in the city. Men living in southern cities with lower HIV prevalence than San Francisco, however, might have had less exposure to HIV and AIDS media awareness campaigns, or targeted prevention information, or both. Thus, the perceived-risk data gathered in these two different studies, using the same questions, allow us the precious opportunity to compare samples from both an AIDS epicenter and from so-called secondary cities, where the spread of HIV has occurred at a slower rate and at a later point in time.

Two of the four questions assessed participants' general concern about AIDS. The first question was, "In comparison to your daily concerns, how concerned are you about AIDS?" This was to be answered in a 10-point scale from *Not at All Concerned* (1) to *Extremely Concerned* (10). In the second question, participants were asked to complete the following statement, "On a normal day, do you think about AIDS . . ." with one of the following responses: *not at all? rarely? once or twice at certain times? on and off through the day? all of the time?*

In both studies, Latino gay and bisexual men showed a great deal of concern and daily preoccupation with AIDS, in comparison to their other daily concerns. To the first question, 43% of the participants in the southern states study and 38% of the participants in the San Francisco study responded with the maximum concern score, a 10 *(Extremely concerned)*. Seventy-four percent of men in southern cities and 71% of men in San Francisco responded with scores of 7 or greater in the 1 to 10 concern score.

The other two questions assessed respondents' estimates about their present and future chances of being infected with HIV. The first question asked, "What do you think are your chances of having the AIDS virus already?" (In San Francisco: "What do you think are your chances of being HIV positive?") Respondents were to choose between *None, Low, Medium, High or Already have HIV* (in San Francisco: *I know I am HIV positive*). Twenty-one percent of men in the southern states study and 25% of men in San Francisco reported knowing that they are already HIV positive. The most striking finding, however, was the low number of men who saw themselves free of risk. Only 20% of men in the South and 10% of men in San Francisco were able to respond with confidence that there was no chance that they were infected at the time of the interview. Interestingly, and contrary to expectations, men in the southern states indicated that their current risk for being HIV positive was higher than the San Francisco men: 34% of the southern men but only 17% of men in San Francisco expressed that their chances of being HIV positive were medium or high.

If we add the number of men who already know they are HIV positive and the number of men who believe their chances of being positive is medium to high, the data from both studies (54% of men in the southern study and 42% in San Francisco) show a great deal of awareness and knowledge about their risk for HIV infection. Because risk behavior (i.e., unprotected anal intercourse) was reported by approximately 50% of Latino gay and bisexual men within a one-year period, the findings from this question suggest that men in both an AIDS epicenter as well as in secondary cities are realistically aware of their risk for HIV. The probable HIV prevalence of 42% for San Francisco is very close to the Department of Health's actual estimate (43%) of HIV infection in Latino gay and bisexual men in the city. If the Department of Health's 43% estimate is correct, and our data (25% reported being HIV positive) represent the population, it means that close to half of the infected men in San Francisco do not know their HIV-positive status. However, taking sampling limitations into account and the absence of data comparing self-report with actual blood testing, this suggests must be considered with great caution.

The fourth and last perceived-risk question asked participants from both studies was to estimate their chances of becoming HIV positive in the future: "What do you think are your own chances of getting the AIDS virus in the future?" (In San Francisco: "What do you think are your chances of becoming HIV positive in the future?") This question was asked only to men who did not say in the previous question that they already knew they were HIV positive. Similar to the previous question, respondents had to state their estimated chance as *none, low, medium,* or *high.* Once again, a very low percentage of men in both studies indicated that their chances were none, 16% in southern cities and 12% in San Francisco. Alarmingly, 40% of men in the southern states study indicated that their future chance of becoming infected with HIV was medium or high; in San Francisco, this percentage was lower (26%) but nonetheless substantial.

In summary, the data just reviewed suggest that Latino gay and bisexual men in the U.S. are not only seriously concerned about the impact of the AIDS epidemic in their lives but also well aware of the personal risks for HIV infection involved in the practice of unprotected sex. Of special concern is the fact that very few men in both samples regarded their risk as zero or none. In fact, large numbers of men believe that there is a considerable (medium to high) chance that they are now or will become infected with HIV in the future. At this time it is not clear whether these findings represent accurate estimates of personal risk, a certain fatalism regarding the inevitability of HIV infection, or a deep mistrust of the actual protective ability of condoms. It is also not clear why men in southern states seem to estimate their HIV risk as higher than do men in San Francisco, contrary to what would be expected. This latter finding could be explained by the fact that many Latino gay and bisexual men (52%) in southern states agreed with the statement, "No matter what you do, no sex is safe." Unfortunately, comparable data are not available for the San Francisco sample.

In any case, what seems crystal clear is that the high frequencies of unprotected anal intercourse in our community, reported in Chapter 1, cannot be explained simply by men's lack of AIDS and HIV awareness or their low perception of personal risk. The perception of high levels of risk does not seem to protect these men from engaging in unprotected sexual practices. Moreover, their perceptions of personal risk seem to correspond quite accurately to, and even go a little higher than, the levels of unprotected sex reported.

Safer Sex Intentions

Most psychological models of behavior change regard the personal formulation of behavioral intentions (e.g., the intention to use condoms in sexual intercourse) as the most important step in changing risk behavior or in adopting new, healthier behavior. In fact, most behavioral models as well as many leading theoreticians assume that, if intentions are strong enough, protective or less risky behavior will most likely follow (see NIMH's Theoreticians' Workshop, Fishbein et al., 1991). Some well-established behavioral models in the health domain, such as the "Theory of Reasoned Action," are mostly concerned with explaining and predicting the formulation of intentions to perform or abstain from a given behavior. It is therefore important to review what we know about safer sex intentions among Latino gay and bisexual men.

I have recently conducted two studies that explicitly assess the existence and strength of personal intentions regarding safer sex among Latino gay and bisexual men in the U.S. The first is the study of 159 Latino men recruited from gay bars in Tucson, Arizona (Díaz et al., 1996); the second is the study of 109 San Francisco gay and bisexual men, recruited conveniently through media advertising, bar outreach, and word of mouth for participation in "El Ambiente," an HIV risk-reduction intervention funded by the city's Department of Health AIDS Office and directed by Dr. Eduardo Morales. The data from El Ambiente I am about to report were collected as a pretest or baseline, prior to the intervention. The data from both studies are limited, however, by the fact that participants were for the most part highly acculturated, English-speaking Latinos.

In both the Tucson and El Ambiente studies, we asked two questions regarding personal intentions to perform safer sex. In Tucson, we asked respondents to express their agreement with the following two statements: "If I'm going to have anal sex, I'm going to use a rubber," and "I have made a commitment to only have anal intercourse with a condom." Responses were scored on a 6-point scale from *Strongly Disagree* to *Strongly Agree*. In San Francisco, we converted the items into questions: "If you are going to have anal sex, are you going to use a condom (rubber)?" and "Have you made a commitment to have anal intercourse only if you use a condom?" Responses were scored on a 4-point scale from *Definitely No* to *Definitely Yes*. While both statements or questions assess the level of personal intentions regarding condom use in anal intercourse, the second statement/question goes further by assessing the presence of an explicit personal commitment to the practice of safer sex.

Analyses of the data from the two studies showed that the majority of men surveyed in Tucson and San Francisco have relatively strong intentions to perform safer sex. In Tucson, the means (sample averages) for the two questions were 5.51 and 5.11 respectively, on a scale where a score of 6 means *Strongly Agree*, indicating the strongest possible intention. When we combined the two items, where a maximum score of 12 indicates the strongest level of intention, we found that 80% of the sample had scores of 10 or above. A similar picture of relatively strong intentions emerged in San Francisco. The means for the two questions were 3.62 and 3.21, on a scale where a score of 4 means *Definitely Yes*, the strongest possible level intention. On a composite score for the two questions, where scores of 6 to 8 indicate affirmative responses to both questions about intentions, we found an average score of 6.9.

In San Francisco, however, the proportion of men that reported the strongest commitment to safer sex was less impressive than expected. In this city, only 78% of respondents said *Definitely Yes* to the first question about using condoms if they have anal sex, and only 67% of respondents said *Definitely Yes* to the question regarding the explicit commitment to have anal sex only if using a condom. The fact that 33% of the men in the San Francisco study were not able to state with certainty that they have made a commitment to safer sex is a bit troublesome.

In support of models of behavior change, it is important to note that the strength of safer sex intentions, as measured in the two studies, did reliably distinguish men who were at risk for HIV and those who were not. Not surprisingly, intentions to practice safer sex were significantly weaker in men who reported instances of unprotected anal intercourse during the last 30 days; these men were labeled the *High-Risk* group. In

Tucson, using the combined two-item score with a highest possible score of 12, men in the *High-Risk* group obtained a mean of 9.26, in comparison to a mean of 11.82 for the *Low-Risk* group. In San Francisco, using the two-question combined score with a highest possible score of 8, men in the *High-Risk* group obtained a mean of 4.97 in comparison to a mean of 7.57 for the *Low-Risk* group. The lowest intention score was obtained by the *High-Risk* group in San Francisco for the question about the explicit commitment to safer sex. These men obtained a mean score of 1.97, on a scale of 1 to 4. All the above differences between risk groups were statistically significant.

Another way of assessing the relationship between safer sex intentions and the actual practice of safer sex among Latino gay and bisexual men is to examine the differential percentages of men, from *High-* and *Low-Risk* groups, who responded with the maximum strength possible (i.e., *Strongly Agree* or *Definitely Yes*) to questions about safer sex intentions. In San Francisco, for example, only 41% of the men in the *High-Risk* group but 91% of the *Low-Risk* group responded *Definitely Yes* to the first question about intentions to use condom. Moreover, only 19% of the men in the *High-Risk* group but 87% of the men in the *Low-Risk* group responded *Definitely Yes* to the question about the explicit commitment to safer sex. These data indicate that stating an explicit and strong commitment to practice safer sex is strongly related to the actual practice of safer sex in the last 30 days. Even though a large proportion (33%) of men did not report a strong commitment to safer sex, the connection between intended behavior and actual practice was quite strong for men in San Francisco.

In summary, the data on safer sex intentions obtained from two different studies suggest that, as a group, Latino gay and bisexual men have relatively strong intentions to practice safer sex or, more specifically, to use condoms during anal intercourse. Of special concern is the fact that men in San Francisco showed weaker levels of intention than men in Tucson, however these inter-city differences might simply reflect the artifactual effects of methodological factors such as the wording of the questions or the response scales used. While not showing a perfect one-to-one relation, the data suggest that intentions are indeed connected to actual condom use in these two groups of highly acculturated Latino gay and bisexual men. Not surprisingly, men who are not practicing safer sex showed weaker personal intentions than their safer peers. In other words, the presence of a strongly and explicitly stated commitment to the practice of safer sex appears as a protective factor against risky sexual behavior. However, as will be discussed in both the next section and in Chapter 4, the relation between intention and behavior is rather fluid and far from perfectly consistent.

The Enactment of Safer Sex Intentions

Because studies have shown that approximately 50% of Latino gay and bisexual men practice unprotected anal intercourse within a period of one year (and about 40% within a period of six months), the relatively strong intentions reported above do not seem to guarantee the maintenance of safer sex behavior over time. Of special importance is to identify those factors (social, psychological, and contextual) that might weaken safer sex intentions or simply break down the intentional, volitional aspects of sexual activity in those Latino gay men who report engaging in unprotected intercourse.

In search of explanations beyond knowledge, perceived risk, and intentions, research has been conducted to examine the "determinants" or "predictors" of HIV risk behavior in Latino gay and bisexual men. To be defined as a predictor of risk, a variable must show a statistically significant correlation with risk behavior, or rates of the given predictor variable should be significantly different in groups who differ in risk behavior. The analysis of differential rates of safer sex intentions for *Low-* and *High-Risk* groups described in the previous section is a concrete example of an analysis of predictors of HIV risk.

As of this writing, only three studies of Latino gay and bisexual men have included quantitative analyses on potential predictors of HIV risk. One of the studies was done with 200 Mexican gay and bisexual men in the Mexico-U.S. border city of Juarez (Ramírez et al., 1994). This study found that unprotected intercourse was significantly more frequent in individuals who (a) were older; (b) were blue-collar (factory) workers; (c) met their partners in streets and places other than gay bars and discos; and (d) had a history of at least one sexually transmitted disease. Because older, blue collar men who prefer anonymous sexual encounters are typically men "in the closet," Ramírez's findings suggest a strong relation between closet issues and HIV risk among men who are Spanish-speaking, of lower socioeconomic status, and perhaps not well integrated as participants in the gay community. Interestingly, the finding that older men in Juarez were at higher risk is both surprising and culturally relevant, given the fact that HIV risk behavior has been found to be more frequent among younger men in studies of White gay men (Stall et al., 1992).

A second set of findings regarding predictors of HIV risk is found in a study of 182 mostly self-identified gay and bisexual Puerto Rican men in New York City (Carballo-Diéguez and Dolezal, 1995). The study found a strong correlation between the practice of unprotected receptive anal intercourse and history of sexual abuse in childhood. According to respondents' reports of sexual activity in childhood, Carballo-Diéguez divided the sample into three groups: (1) *Abuse* group, men who before the age of 13 had sex with a partner at least four years older and who felt hurt by the experience or were unwilling to participate in it; (2) *Willing/not hurt* group—men who had an older partner before age 13 but did not feel hurt by the experience and were willing to participate; and (3) *No older partner* group. The study found a clear and strong linear relationship between history of sexual abuse and HIV risk: 56% of the abused group, 42% of the willing/not hurt group, and 22% of the *No older partner* group reported having recently engaged in the practice of unprotected receptive anal intercourse.

More recently, in the study of 159 men recruited from gay bars in Tucson, Díaz et al. (1996) analyzed differences between High and Low HIV-risk groups along different psychosocial variables. Two cognitive variables (safer sex intentions and self-perceptions of sexual control) and two behavioral variables (sex under the influence of drugs, alcohol, or both, and anonymous sex in public places) were significantly different in Low and High HIV-risk groups. Men who had practiced unprotected anal intercourse with a non-monogamous partner during the previous month had (a) weaker intentions to practice safer sex; (b) lower perceptions of sexual control; (c) more instances of sex while intoxicated; and (d) a higher frequency of anonymous sexual encounters in public sex environments. The two behavioral predictors of risk suggest that risky behavior may occur in situations where the sexual activity of Latino gay and bisexual men is disconnected from personal conscious control (through the influence of alcohol and drugs) and disconnected from interpersonal relations and interaction and negotiation (through anonymous sex in public environments).

In summary, the relatively small number of studies that have analyzed predictors or determinants of HIV risk in Latino gay and bisexual men have yielded a wealth of information regarding the factors—cognitive, developmental, behavioral, and contextual—that might weaken men's intentions and commitment to behave in a sexually safer manner. Closet issues in the face of pervasive homophobia, coupled with painful experiences and memories of childhood sexual abuse, may contribute to a sexuality that is disconnected from a sense of personal control and interpersonal/affective relations. The disconnection of sexuality from interpersonal, affective, and volitional processes, and the accompanying perceptions of low sexual control, might be exacerbated by the abusive use of drugs and alcohol during sexual activity. The predictors of risk from behavioral research, however, point to the role of deeper sociocultural factors in the risk of HIV, such as machismo, homophobia, and sexual silence, that have shaped developmentally, and needless to say oppressively, the sexuality of Latino men who experience same-sex desire. The next few chapters will explore with more detail those factors that weaken the enactment of safer sex intentions.

Summary and Conclusions

In summary, behavioral research done to date converges on the following findings:

1. Approximately 50% of Latino gay and bisexual men in the U.S., within a period of one year, practice unprotected anal intercourse, a behavior that represents one of the highest risk factors for the transmission of HIV.

2. Risk behavior continues to occur in the presence of substantial knowledge about HIV and AIDS, accurate perceptions of personal risk, and relatively strong intentions to practice safer sex.

3. Knowledge about HIV and AIDS, however, is not perfect. There is a need for continued education on matters related to modes of HIV transmission and means of prevention, especially specific information regarding proper and satisfying condom use. Furthermore, there is evidence that condom use might be undermined by a widespread belief that "no sex is ever safe." Information campaigns should especially target those men who are at "the fringes" of gay

community, such as Spanish-speaking men of low socioeconomic status, those who are recent immigrants, youths, and those who are forced to remain in the homophobic closet.

4. Strong intentions to practice safer sex, such as the presence of an explicit personal commitment to use condoms in sexual intercourse, play an important protective role against risky sexual behavior. There is evidence, however, that safer sex intentions can be seriously weakened by cognitive (e.g., a perception of low sexual control), behavioral (e.g., sex while intoxicated), and contextual (e.g., sex in public sex environments) factors that disconnect or dissociate sexual activity from conscious volitional and interpersonal regulatory process.

5. HIV risk in Latino gay and bisexual men is strongly associated with closet issues, sex under the influence of alcohol and drugs, anonymous sex in public places, and low perceptions of sexual control. These determinants of risk might be fostered and exacerbated by the devastating, yet often unrecognized, effects of childhood sexual abuse in many members of our community.

Even though the behavioral studies done to date provide a wealth of information regarding the situation of Latino gay and bisexual men and the risk for HIV, our knowledge is quite limited on a number of fronts. I would like to list some of these important gaps in our knowledge as suggestions for further research.

1. With very few exceptions, the overwhelming majority of study participants to date have been English-speaking, highly acculturated, Latino gay and bisexual men. It is not clear whether the findings reported in this review can be generalized reliably to men who are Spanish-speaking, of low socioeconomic status, and not well integrated to the mainstream community. We need systematic research where variables relevant to HIV prevention in Latino gay and bisexual men are studied as a function of acculturation or integration into the mainstream, English-speaking gay community.

2. With only three studies of predictors of risk to date, there exists a dire need for more systematic analyses of predictors or determinants of unprotected intercourse in our community, beyond those variables suggested by psychological models of behavior change. In par-

ticular, there is a need to investigate determinants of risk in light of underlying sociocultural factors. The identification of important sociocultural predictors of risk will help us develop interventions to reduce HIV risk in a well-focused, effective, and culturally relevant manner.

3. A big gap remains between qualitative and quantitative research in the area, where both types of research are being conducted in a parallel, non-interacting fashion. There is an urgent need to construct quantitative surveys based on the actual subjective experiences of Latino gay and bisexual men, as voiced in the qualitative study of narratives. Conversely, there is a need to conduct more qualitative, in-depth research on those variables identified as important predictors of risk by quantitative research, such as experiences of childhood sexual abuse, the use of intoxicants during sex, and the perceptions of low sexual control.

4. Finally, to date there are no published HIV risk-reduction interventions targeted at Latino gay and bisexual men that have been carefully and scientifically evaluated for their effectiveness in promoting the use of condoms and safer sex. There is an urgent need to develop, implement, and evaluate culturally relevant interventions based on our knowledge to date. It is my hope that this book will promote the development and careful evaluation of such interventions.

3.

Cultural Barriers
to Behavior Change

As discussed in the last chapter, quantitative studies of Latino gay and bisexual men in the U.S. have revealed a positive correlation between individuals' intentions to practice safer sex and their reported condom use in sexual encounters. Not surprisingly, individuals who use protection consistently tend to report stronger intentions and personal commitments to practice safer sex than do individuals who engage in risky sexual behavior. Although the relationship is statistically significant, however, intention to practice safer sex tends to be a weak predictor of behavior in this population, explaining in some studies only about 3% of the variance in reported condom use (see, e.g., Díaz et al., 1996). The fact remains that a substantial number of study participants who were not protecting themselves have also reported personal plans, strong intentions, and explicit commitments to use condoms for HIV prevention. The fact that a personal intention to practice safer sex may coexist with the practice of unprotected or unsafe sexual behavior is not only psychologically puzzling but also in need of further explanation.

Understanding the variables that compete with the enactment of relatively strong personal intentions in the practice of safer sex is crucial to the task of HIV prevention. If "weaker" intentions are indeed a significant predictor of unsafe sexual practices, our task is then to understand the factors that weaken such intentions. Moreover, repeated failure to enact personal intentions leads to a sense of helplessness and fatalism that undermines perceived self-efficacy and negatively affects the formulation, strength, and enactment of future intentions (Bandura, 1994).

For two important reasons, an explanation of intention-behavior relations is particularly pressing for the field of HIV prevention research. First, a large number of theories of behavior change in the field have focused on the processes by which individuals come to formulate behavioral intentions, rather than on the processes and circumstances by which the intentions can or cannot be enacted. Second, there is substantial evidence that a number of interpersonal (e.g., peer pressure, sexual coercion, threat of rejection) as well as personal (e.g., decreased pleasure, sexual discomfort, a pressing need for intimate contact and connection) variables compete rather strongly with the enactment of well-meaning safer sex intentions, as formulated by sexually active individuals who are considered at risk for HIV infection.

I have written this chapter in order to introduce the main thesis of the book, namely, that sociocultural variables, or internalized cultural scripts, might indeed interfere with the enactment of safer sex intentions and behavior change. I have organized the chapter into three major sections. The first section presents a critique of current models of behavior change, especially those Western psychological and health models that assume individual, cognitive, volitional control over sexual behavior. The second section, based on qualitative data on Latino gay men, describes sociocultural factors that regulate sexual behavior and shed light on person-situation contexts that undermine the enactment of safer sex intentions. In the last and third section, based on findings to date, I propose three hypotheses that might explain the HIV risk of Latino gay men from their unique sociocultural perspective. Chapters 4, 5, and 6 will elaborate the identified cultural barriers with greater detail, particularly by bringing the voices and subjective experiences of Latino gay men to the forefront of the discussion.

Models of Behavior Change for HIV Prevention

The overwhelming majority of HIV prevention research in the U.S. has been guided by a limited set of relatively well-known "models of behavior change": Health Belief Model; Theory of Reasoned Action; AIDS Risk Reduction Model (ARRM); Prochaska and DiClemente's Stages of Change; Bandura's Social Cognitive Theory, and, more recently, Fisher and Fisher's Information-Motivation-Skills (I-M-S) model of HIV risk behavior. These models have been useful and productive on many different counts. For example, perceived self-efficacy, as postulated by Bandura, has emerged as a significant predictor of sexual risk behavior in most studies that have measured the variable (Coates et al., 1988). Similarly, recent analyses by Fisher and Fisher (1994) have documented their model's ability to predict 35% of the variance in the sexual risk behavior reported by a sample of gay males (the same model, however, predicted only 10% of risk behavior variance in heterosexual college students).

As theoretical guides for HIV prevention research and interventions, however, the majority of these models are seriously limited on three different fronts:

1. With the exception of the ARRM and Fisher and Fisher's I-M-S, the models were originally formulated for domains other than sexuality and drug use, and in contexts other than HIV prevention.
2. Models typically emphasize and were designed to predict the personal formulation of individuals' behavioral intentions, with little attention to the contexts and situations where intentions must be enacted.
3. Even though many of the models give some weight to the impact of social norms on individuals' behavior, they assume that the behavior in question is under individual volitional control. In other words, the models assume that if individuals' intentions are strong enough, behavior will follow:

In an integrating "Theorist's Workshop" sponsored by the National Institute of Mental Health (Fishbein et al., 1991), a group of influential American theorists explored points of both convergence and debate in their efforts to understand behavior prediction and behavior change within the context of HIV prevention. Early on in the workshop's report, the theorists underscored two major points of consensus or agreement.

The first point of agreement was that AIDS transmission is a consequence of an individual's behavior:

AIDS is first and foremost a consequence of behavior. It is *not who you are, but what you do* that determine(s) whether or not you expose yourself to HIV, the virus that causes AIDS. (p. 1; italics added)

While justly attempting to move away from biased notions regarding HIV transmission based on membership to "risk groups," the theorists went to another biased extreme. By locating the causes of HIV transmission in individual behavior, the theorists moved away from structural or cultural analyses of human behavior, where sexual behavior can be understood as regulated by sociocultural, political, and economic structures, especially the power structures that shape and determine gender-appropriate norms and behavior (see, e.g., Amaro, 1995).

Interestingly, the theorists defined AIDS transmission within the context of individual behavior even when clear epidemiological data in the U.S. locate the virus not randomly distributed across the population but in specific contexts defined by social experiences of poverty, racism, and homophobia within minority populations (NCA, 1992). It is precisely in those contexts where a sense of socially imposed powerlessness and fatalism, among others things, seriously limit individuals' ability to enact personal intentions. In other words, the HIV-prevention theorists seemed to overlook the fact that "who you are," defined by your particular sociocultural context, explains and determines to a great extent what you can and cannot do.

The second point of agreement in the theorists' workshop was that if a personal intention is strong enough, behavior will follow:

> There was general consensus that the intention to perform a given behavior is one of the immediate determinants of that behavior. The stronger one's intention to perform a given behavior, the greater the likelihood that the person will, in fact, perform that behavior. (p. 5)

Even though this statement does have certain validity for many individuals or groups, the reality is that in many individuals, risky behavior does co-exist with relatively strong intentions to act safely and promote one's health. It is my belief that intentions lead to behavior only in situations where individuals have power and control over the consequences of their behavior, or when individuals have enough resources to deal with negative outcomes or consequences as a result of enacting their intentions. Unfortunately, this is not the case for those groups where HIV is spreading at faster rates in this country: gay men of color, minority women, the young, the poor.

It should be noted that the positive correlations between intention and behavior noted above were found mostly among groups of highly acculturated, English-speaking, Latino gay and bisexual men. Those same studies revealed a strong relationship between risky sexual behavior and socioeconomic markers of income and education within the samples (Díaz et al., 1996).

By placing the causes of HIV transmission in individual behavior, the theorists biased the focus of prevention toward individual responsibility (so true to the American tradition!), minimizing the role of structural and sociocultural determinants. Not surprisingly, with few exceptions, theories proposed to date have overlooked the processes— personal, interpersonal, and situational—involved in the enactment of intentions within the context of multiple competing factors, including low perceptions of personal control and a sense of fatalism regarding the inevitability of infection so ever-present in impoverished, powerless, vulnerable groups. As a consequence, the majority of theories have focused on cognitive and perceptual factors and, for example, have given more weight to individuals' perceptions of control (e.g., perceived self-efficacy) rather than to actual (real world) determinants or limitations of individual control over individual health-promoting decisions and behavior. Finally, these models have given little attention to individual and group differences in the expression of human sexuality or to the cultural determinants of sexual behavior.

There is obviously a need for a shift of paradigm in HIV prevention research. We need to develop models that are domain specific (sexuality and drug use) and that focus on the difficulties that persons, dyads, and communities face in the enactment of personal intentions. More importantly, we need models that focus on the breakdown of intentionality, and that are sensitive to the historical, cultural, situational, and contextual variables where risky sexual behavior occurs. Of special importance would be an attempt to understand risk behavior not in terms of "deficits" in individuals' knowledge, motivation, or skills, but rather as behavior that may have meaning and be quite rational and logical within a given sociocultural context.

Sociocultural Barriers to the Enactment of Safer Sex Intentions

In order to understand the factors that compete with the practice of safer sex, I interviewed approximately 70 Latino gay and bisexual men in San Francisco during the period of November 1992 through June 1993. The majority of participants were interviewed in the context of 10 focus groups; 9 men were interviewed in individual, in-depth interviews. The men were recruited through establishments, organizations, agencies, and friendship networks, ensuring that both Spanish-speaking, non-acculturated men and English-speaking, acculturated men were included. Focus groups and interviews were conducted in either Spanish or English, as appropriate. Approximately half of the sample was Mexican or of Mexican descent; the rest of the sample included eight different nationalities from the Caribbean, Central, and South America. One focus group was done with 5 "Vestidas" ("the ones who dress-up," feminine ending -as), which is the collective name for transvestite and transgender persons within the non-acculturated Latino gay and bisexual community. Another focus group included 5 men who had worked for some time with other gay and bisexual men as health educators and outreach workers within Latino-identified AIDS education and prevention programs in the city.

Focus group and interview questions were formulated to elicit the subjective experiences of Latino gay and bisexual men regarding their developmental and social histories as self-identified gay and bisexual men in Latino communities; their past and current sexual behavior; their perceptions of risk for HIV infection; their level of commitment to practice safer sex; the perceived difficulties and barriers to safe sex practices; and the major sources of social support, including the relationships to their own families and friends, to the Latino community, and to the mainstream gay community in San Francisco.

As expected, men in San Francisco showed a high degree of knowledge about HIV and AIDS, accurate perceptions of risk, and a strong desire to protect themselves and their loved ones and remain healthy. However, in the presence of substantial knowledge, accurate risk perceptions, and positive intentions, the men reported multiple incidents of risky behavior in risky situations, including multiple partners, prostitution, sex in public environments, the use of intoxicants during sexual activity, and instances of unprotected anal intercourse.

The most striking element of the focus group and in-depth interview data was the parallel I found between men's experiences growing up as self-identified but closeted homosexuals in the context of their Latino families, on the one hand, and the expressed difficulties in the practice of safer sex on the other. There were some striking congruences and mean-ingful relationship between the answers given for the following two seem-ingly unrelated questions: "What is it like to be a Latino gay or bisexual man?" and "What is the most difficult aspect of practicing safe sex?"

For example, in response to the first question, men talked about the painful doubts about their masculinity during childhood, doubts raised by a social context where homosexuality is defined as a "gender" prob-lem (i.e., homosexual men are defined as women in men's bodies, or as not being "real" men) rather than sexual orientation. Men talked about the need to prove their masculinity in order to feel accepted by other boys and to participate in an often cruel peer culture. In parallel fash-ion, in response to the second question, men talked about the fear of losing their erections when using condoms and appearing less than manly or like a *loca* (cultural equivalent of "queen"). Men often described sexual encounters as events where they could show their masculinity, or experience the masculinity of their partners through dominant, strong, penetrative practices. For many of these men, through important developmental experiences, sexuality has been con-structed as a place to create and restore a sense of masculinity and macho ideal. Thus, an extreme focus on penetration and fear of losing erections, identified as major barriers to safer sex, became clearly mean-ingful within the sociocultural context of machismo for those men who experience same-sex desires within Latino communities.

Similar parallels between internalized sociocultural values and high-risk practices were found for other identified risk factors. For example, there was a clear and meaningful connection between the fact that too often family acceptance of homosexuality can be achieved only through silence ("They know but we can't talk about it"), and the problems men had in talking about sexuality or negotiating safer sex. The strong and prevalent perception that homosexuality "hurts my family" was closely related to a sense of sexual shame and a separation of sexuality and social, interpersonal, and affective life as manifested by frequent sexual activity within the context of hidden encounters with strangers in pub-lic cruising environments.

The focus group data showed that, among most Latino gay and bisexual men interviewed, unsafe practices were not the product of a "deficit" in AIDS knowledge, motivation, or skills. Rather, important sociocultural factors and values (by now internalized through socialization practices and currently reinforced by participation in Latino communities and family life) strongly compete with the enactment of safer sex intentions.

Based on the San Francisco findings, I have outlined a set of barriers or competing factors to the enactment of safer sex intentions. The barriers are listed under six different headings with the assumption that they are expressions of six internalized sociocultural factors. Thus, the barriers are seen not as personal deficits or shortcomings, but rather as logical outcomes or specific manifestations of socialization processes in the sexual lives of Latino gay and bisexual men.

Machismo

(A) an extreme and almost exclusive focus on penetrative sexual practices to the extent that sex without penetration is not considered sex;
(B) perceptions of low sexual control, where a state of high sexual arousal (*estar caliente*; "being hot") is used as a socially-accepted justification for unprotected sex and the surrender of reflective/regulatory control in sexual encounters; and
(C) a perception of sexuality as a favored place to prove masculinity, where the possibility of losing penile erection is avoided at all costs.

Homophobia

(A) a strong sense of personal shame about same-sex sexual desire, so much so that fear of rejection in sexual encounters takes precedence over health concerns;
(B) serious problems in self-identification as a member of a group at risk, with consequent denial of personal vulnerability to HIV; and
(C) feelings of anxiety about same-sex sexual encounters, leading to an increased use of alcohol, drugs, and other intoxicants in preparation for sexual activity.

Family Loyalty
(in the context of close personal involvement with homophobic families)

(A) closeted lives with low levels of identification with and social support from a peer gay community;
(B) minimal influence of normative changes in the gay community on sexual behavior because families are seen as the main social-referent group; and

(C) a forced separation between sexuality and social/affective life or relationships that promotes anonymous, hidden encounters in public cruising places.

Sexual Silence

(A) problems in talking openly about sexuality, resulting in difficulties with sexual communication or safer sex negotiation in sexual encounters;

(B) increased sexual discomfort with all matters pertinent to sexuality; and

(C) the psychological dissociation of sexual thoughts and feelings, decreasing the likelihood of accurate self-observation within the domain of sexuality.

Poverty

(A) decreased sense of personal control over one's life, leading to fatalistic notions regarding health and personal well-being;

(B) increased unemployment, drug abuse, and violence, undermining the consideration of HIV infection as a major, central, or priority concern; and

(C) situations of financial dependence such as living with families, exploitative relations with older men, and prostitution, where the personal power for self-determination and self-regulation is seriously undermined.

Racism

(A) increased personal shame about being Latino, with serious negative consequences on self-esteem and personal identity;

(B) lack of participation in the mainstream gay community and its activities (racist and classist values regarding personal looks, financial power, and educational achievement, highly prevalent in the mostly White and middle-class gay community, conspire against feelings of belonging and social recognition for gay men of color); and

(C) racist stereotypes about Latino men as being "passionate, dark and exotic," creating pressure from non-Latino White gay men to practice risky sex.

While it is possible to identify specific competing factors for any given group of individuals or population, such as "Latino gay men," the strength of the actual competition, that is the degree to which competing variables actually become barriers to the enactment of the intentions, will most likely vary among individuals in the group. For example, if fear of interpersonal rejection competes with the intention to use condoms in a sexual encounter, the actual competing effect of the fear vis-à-vis the enactment of the safer sex intention will vary according to individuals' senses of loneliness and alienation, and their consequent need for human contact, touch, and relationship. This is why it is always important to define competing variables in relation to individuals' needs and meanings within a given sociocultural and interpersonal context.

Moreover, as outlined above, these competing difficulties or "barriers" to the practice of safer sex, whenever possible, should be conceptually linked to the specific cultural context that has shaped the sexual development of the individuals in question. That is, there is a need to examine and make explicit the "cultural lens" by which the particular difficulties are meaningful and logical to the individuals who experience them. For example, it is of paramount importance in this endeavor to examine the powerful effects of gender socialization within the given culture and articulate its relation to both heterosexual and homosexual activity. Similarly, it is important to examine what constitutes the domain of accepted public awareness (e.g., fathers taking adolescent sons to prostitutes in order to "prove their manhood") and, conversely, what is defined by the culture as shameful and secret (e.g., the sexual penetration of young effeminate boys by self-defined heterosexual men).

Only under the light of such a cultural lens can the expressed and observed difficulties in the practice of safer sex be seen as meaningful behavior. Prevention programs aimed at and focused on "changing behavior," but not taking into account such deeply internalized cultural meanings, are doomed to failure.

Three Hypotheses about Latino Gay Men

In preparation for the chapters that follow, I would like to advance three specific hypotheses about the risk for HIV in Latino gay men.

First, given their cultural and sexual socialization, the practice of safer sex is difficult and challenging for Latino gay men, especially in circumstances that challenge or threaten the internalized cultural scripts. For example, if sexuality has been culturally defined as a powerful place to prove masculinity or restore a hurt sense of manhood, contexts and situations that threaten the loss of what is perceived as a virile erection will be extremely challenging and difficult. Similarly, if Latinos are welcome and accepted into the mainstream gay community mostly when acting out a "careless, hot, and passionate" stereotype—to the extent that sexual regulation and control are seen an un-Latino—they will be frequently coerced into risky sexual activity by members of the mainstream culture.

Second, due to diminished opportunities to self-observe in the domain of sexuality, a breakdown of self-regulatory processes is likely to occur for Latino gay men in the face of increasing challenge and difficulty. A necessary condition for the exercise of self-regulation and self-determination in the practice of safer sex is the individual's awareness of the personal, interpersonal, and situational variables that make such behavior difficult, or that compete with the enactment of safer sex intentions. In other words, individuals' capacities for sexual self-regulation are based on their awareness of the "competing variables" and of the difficult contexts to practice safer sex. In Bandura's (1986) social-cognitive model, self-observation stands as the first and most basic sub-function of self-regulation. In his own words, "people cannot influence their own actions very well if they are inattentive to relevant aspects of their behavior.... If they want to exert influence over their actions, they have to know what they are doing" (p. 336).

For the majority of Latino gay men, however, their homosexuality has been culturally accepted (or rather tolerated) only if it is not mentioned or talked about and not labeled as such. In my opinion, the lack of social space to name, speak, share, discuss, and critically reflect about one's homosexual behavior and relations, outside of macho boasting about one's sexual prowess or conquests, has led to a decreased ability to reflect, observe, and consequently regulate our sexual activity. I propose, therefore, that the overwhelming majority of Latino gay men, because of the homophobia and sexual silence of our culture, might not have had the socially supported opportunities to self-observe in the domain of sexuality; in the words of one of my research participants, "we just don't know ourselves sexually." This lack of self-observation may lead to a decreased ability to self-regulate in the sexual domain.

The third hypothesis is that, in light of such volitional, self-regulatory breakdown, *culturally scripted information*, rather than self-formulated intentions or plans of action, become the main regulators and determinants of sexual behavior. In the case of Latino gay men who live in the U.S., I have proposed that the following set of six sociocultural variables or factors—machismo, homophobia, family loyalty, sexual silence, poverty, and racism—constitute the basic forces that give shape to the psycho-cultural scripts that regulate our sexual behavior. Because these six cultural factors explain and give meaning to what appears from the outside as simply "risky behavior," a major claim is that the high occurrence of unprotected sex among Latino gay men has logic and meaning from our given sociocultural perspective.

Whenever possible, in the next three chapters, I will give voice to the men I have interviewed in order to show how the six cultural factors are internalized and subjectively experienced in the context of sexual activity. I will attempt to show that these sociocultural factors, now internalized, have become competing variables or major barriers to the practice of safer sex, and how they weaken self-regulatory or personal control of sexual activity. In particular, I want to show how the experience of such cultural factors has been oppressive, wounding our self-esteem, undermining our perceptions of sexual control, and promoting a certain fatalism about the inevitability of HIV infection.

4.

Machismo and Homophobia

The Wounding of Self-Esteem

They see me with desire
thinking I am "bugarron"
but they are totally wrong . . .
more "hembra" than me
in bed they'll never find.

—"*Me siento lindo y hermoso,*" poem by Tatiana
Perra! La Revista, vol 1, no.2. June–July 1995
(translation by RMD)

Bugarron: Heterosexually identified man who pen-
etrates other men. *Hembra:* A real woman, female
equivalent of macho.

It is impossible to write about the experiences of homophobia in the lives of Latino gay men without addressing cultural ideals about men and masculinity. Homosexual boys are socialized in the context of three messages that link machismo and homophobia in an oppressive partnership. In a single stroke, the messages both inflate our self-concept and destructively wound our dignity and self-esteem.

A first message defines masculinity, the essence of male identity, in terms of highly prized virtues such as courage, fearlessness, protection, and strength. Men are given privileged status as carriers and defenders of cultural treasures—financial, political, social, and psychological. As feminist writers have pointed out, patriarchal societies are organized to maintain male domination, giving males not only access to power but also ample opportunities for asserting and establishing their self-worth and self-esteem. If this were the only message received about our manhood, we would predict that most males in Latino communities, heterosexual and homosexual alike, would grow up with a strong sense of self-assertion and self-esteem, though perhaps pedantic, inflated, and unacceptably oppressive toward women.

A second and perhaps more powerful message is that not all men are masculine and that, in fact, masculinity must be *proven* by exceptional feats of courage, fearlessness and strength. This second message, the need to prove masculinity, breeds restlessness, anxiety, and self-doubt. Masculinity is presented not as a praiseworthy personal virtue but as some kind of northern star that, while ever-present in our personal journey, can never be truly reached.

It is this message that promotes "machismo" or "hypermasculinity," the excessive, abusive, and perverted display of masculine traits, most often in response to personal doubts about achieving the masculine ideal. Deeper doubts and insecurity about one's masculinity, and "non-masculine" feelings of helplessness and fear, predict stronger displays of *machista* attitudes and behavior. It is my belief that the combined message stating "It's great to be a man, but you are not one until you prove it" constitutes a powerful predictor and explains much of the behavior as well as many of the psychological characteristics and emotional wounds attributed to Latino males—homosexuals not excepted.

The third message, most devastating for Latino gay men, states that "homosexuals are not true men" or, even worse, "homosexuals are *failed* men." In our culture, as in many others, homosexuality has been defined in terms of gender identity rather than sexual orientation (Almaguer, 1991); that is, homosexuals are not considered true or real men—"*no hombres hombres*"—as one research participant told me with great emphasis and conviction. Homosexuality in men is conceived as the failure to achieve the culturally given and highly prized masculine ideal and, therefore, is something to scorn and be ashamed of. While femininity is socially regarded as desired virtue in women and defined "in contrast to" or "in complement to" masculinity in men, those same feminine characteristics in males, including same-sex attraction, are understood and regarded by the culture as shameful personal failures. The stronger and deeper the machismo ideology in a given community, the more homophobic attitudes can be expected.

The definition of homosexuality as a gender problem rather than as a difference in sexual orientation fuels and exacerbates homophobia. Homosexuals are portrayed in terms of those characteristics that must be avoided precisely by those involved in proving masculinity. It is no surprise that the most common insult among boys who are working out their sense of manhood among other boys is *maricón,* the cultural equivalent of "faggot." Homosexuals carry the burden of portraying and embodying the "failure scenario," a reminder of masculinity gone wrong. Homosexuals thus serve as the target of anger, violence, and disgust, like a perverted support system for boys' insecurities in their task of proving manhood. It is no wonder that many boys who experience same-sex desire end up in silence, highly inhibited, and feeling that they are wearing a false mask of masculinity.

Because of the culture's definition of homosexuality in terms of gender identification rather than sexual orientation, boys who experience same-sex desires tend to be tortured with doubt about their masculinity. The machismo triple message is, therefore, perceived as particularly relevant and accusatory by homosexual boys, leading to a more pronounced need to prove effortfully their masculinity. Some boys, especially those with more effeminate characteristics, may give up early on in their attempts to prove manhood and may construct a feminine identification. Others, less extreme, grow up believing that they are not truly *"hombres hombres"* (men men) or "real men" like their heterosexual counterparts, constructing the idea that their masculinity is in reality a show or facade that hides more or less successfully the *loca* (crazy woman, cultural equivalent of "queen") within. Effeminate homosexuals are referred to as "obvious," meaning that all homosexuals are deep down effeminate and womanlike, and what varies among us is the degree of our concealment.

Thus, even though it may appear somewhat counterintuitive, my working hypothesis is that gay-identified men who grow up in Latino cultures are more vulnerable to the machismo message and, therefore, would be more concerned and compelled to prove their masculinity than their heterosexual peers. For those who understandably give up proving their own manhood, the cultural message of machismo often turns into an obsession to experience the manhood of their sexual partners, to the point of feeling sexually attracted only to straight or straight-looking men.

A Personal Story

It took me at least six months to finally produce some writing on the topic of this chapter. Time and time again, I approached the keyboard only to become paralyzed with a familiar, empty, painful feeling in the stomach—that very same feeling evoked by the recess bell during my school years in Cuba, Guatemala, and Puerto Rico.

While my classmates expressed joy and relief, the bell signaled for me another half-hour of name calling—*Pato, Pajarito, Mariquita, Maricón*—and, quite often, physical abuse. As the unwilling subject of an ill-fated Pavlovian experiment, the recess bell produced in me a certain anticipatory panic for the forthcoming laughs, name calling, threats, punches, and kicks, all of these woven into some kind of message about my failed masculinity. At recess time, being left alone was a most welcome though bittersweet relief. I wanted so much to be approached, included, and respected by other boys! But solitude was much better than never-ending harassment.

Very puzzling at the time was the fact that when many other boys at my school were called the colorful variety of "faggot" names, they either casually returned the insults, jokingly fought back, or seemed to have cared less. Much to my confusion and surprise, many classmates shrugged off the name calling and acted as if the terrifying insults bounced off their very tough skins. It was clear to me that the wide variety of faggot insults were not only directed at me; in fact, with few exceptions, everyone got their share.

But I reacted differently. Unlike the seemingly casual, transitory, and only skin-deep effects on my peers, the insults tortured me and left me paralyzed in a combination of panic and despair. I believed somehow the insults contained a kernel of truth. The insults were validated, in my mind, by the emerging awareness of my own homosexuality. In fact, more than being insulted, it felt like I was being publicly and shamefully *exposed*. In those days, I had recurrent dreams of shame, such as finding myself in my underwear, right in the middle of the school playground full of kids.

At recess time, I was not only a victim but also my most severe and damaging perpetrator. I tortured myself with questions of personal doubt: Was it my voice? Was it the way I moved my hands? Was it my terror and deep aversion to violence? My dislike of rough sports? Or was it that unexplainable feeling of weakness in my arms that made me physically unable to punch my insulting opponent in self-defense? I grew up with the disturbing conclusion that there was something profoundly wrong with me. After all, I felt in the most profound physical guttural ways, those shameful feelings the faggot names described.

My shame, though obviously connected to my sexual feelings, was more clearly focused on failed masculinity. More deeply shameful than sex was the fear that I was publicly failing at the most important task or sacred ideal—manhood—given to me by family, media, and peers. I had learned very well what a man should feel, say, and do, and I knew I couldn't feel, say, and do it that way. I felt in my gut the despair of someone who could not reach what seemed, at first view, a very simple goal, a goal apparently reached by everyone else around me with relatively little effort. I felt, and knew, that I could not be what I was supposed to be, "a real man," as dictated by my culture. I remember dreaming exhausting dreams of constant walking, running, climbing, never able to reach the place, the finish line, the summit. My mother told me once, in recent years, that as a child I complained a lot of being tired. My parents thought it was my flat feet; now, I know better. At the time, however, my flat feet were yet another confirmation, as concrete as they come, that there was something profoundly wrong with me.

Thoughts of denial and escape, at different levels of self-awareness, provided some welcome relief. After all, the sex stuff could be kept in secret or maybe eventually changed if I had sex with a female prostitute, or kissed a girlfriend, or married a woman some day. I was a sensual, sexual, passionate child and remember enjoying thoroughly a woman's touch and affection. I remember getting aroused by anything sexual, even magazines of naked women or older boys' tales of heterosexual prowess. Of course, so I thought, I could become a celibate priest and store my sexuality safely in a locked drawer—all of which I did for a number of years—so I could live happily ever after with pride and respect from my family and friends. But there was not much relief for that feeling of deficiency, for that sense of personal weakness and failure with respect to the culture's masculine ideal.

At age 46, as an openly gay man, with years of participation in the gay liberation movement, and a 10-year veteran of psychotherapy, I had no idea it would be so difficult to write about the impact of machismo and homophobia. But now I realize that, in so doing, I am revisiting and exploring the origins of the most profound wounds I carry. In fact, I could not have written this chapter except by telling at one point my personal story and recognizing my personal wounds.

This chapter is about me and men like me who grew up homosexual in Latino communities, where an intricate alliance between machismo and homophobia has devoured our sense of dignity and self-esteem, in the same way that HIV is now devouring our immune systems. I believe that the experiences of machismo and homophobia, and their destructive linkage in our culture, hold the most important clues to understanding what is happening to us and our sexuality. This chapter is thus an exploration of those forces that have told me and other Latino gay men like me that there is something wrong with us. It is a journey into the sources of profound restlessness and shame, and the underlying reason why many of us have always overachieved with a sense that it is never good enough.

In retrospect, I am fully aware that the damaging effects of machismo and homophobia were possible not only because we have been the object of substantial verbal and physical abuse, but mainly because *we have seen ourselves with the same eyes as our oppressors*. Therefore, this chapter is more about internalized machismo and homophobia, about internalized oppression, rather than about machismo and homophobia in our culture, objectively defined as external to us. I embark on this exploration with a great deal of hope and conviction that healing our self-esteem—through proud self-affirmation—is indeed possible.

Homosexuality as a Gender Category

The most destructive link between the messages of machismo and homophobia is achieved by a cultural definition of homosexuality as a gender problem, rather than a difference in sexual orientation. Homosexuals are defined as not real men, as less than men or, more appropriately, as failed men. *Maricón*, the culturally equivalent word for *faggot*, denounces those who are effeminate, those who fail the masculinity test.

As socialized members of the culture, many Latino homosexuals, especially those who have not been touched by gay liberation ideology, share this oppressive, homophobic cultural definition. An extreme preoccupation with masculinity/femininity of self and sexual partners, a personal sense of shame for being or appearing effeminate, and the frequent adoption of an internal and external feminine identity, are just a few of the many manifestations of such self-oppressive ideology. Even though many Latino gay men have creatively and humorously dealt with the cultural definition of failed manhood, "My family loved me, I was the princess of the house" or "We were five, I mean, four-and-a-half, brothers"—in my opinion, this internalization constitutes and continues to be one of the most devastating wounds to our self-esteem. The end product is a pervasive feeling, often quite vague and diffuse, that something is deeply wrong with us.

Nowhere is the interpretation of homosexuality as a gender category so obvious as in a poem entitled *"Me siento lindo y hermoso"* (I feel pretty and beautiful), written for a Spanish-speaking gay audience in Miami. The poem provides us with a clear example of a gay man who, while he doesn't dress up as a woman or aspire for a sex change, has internalized and adopted society's gender definition of homosexuality. Indeed, the most interesting and intriguing aspect of the poem is that it was written by a gay man using the pseudonym *Tatiana*, for *Perra!* magazine (note the feminine names for both author and publication) for an audience of mostly Latino gay men. It is far from being considered an insult. According to Eduardo Aparico, editor of *Perra!* magazine, the poem's author intends to mock and ridicule the machista attitude or "masculine façade" displayed by many Latino homosexuals. The poem witnesses the depth of acceptance and internalization of a gender definition of homosexuality in our community. This occurs apparently with little awareness that this perspective effectively links, in an oppressive manner, machismo and homophobia in our culture.

The poem was originally written in Spanish and, on the right side, I offer my translation.

Me siento lindo y hermoso	I feel pretty and beautiful
porque estoy bien musculoso.	because I am so muscular.
Pero las locas no saben	But the queens don't know
que entre las piernas hay poco.	there is little between my legs.
Me miran con ilusión,	They see me with desire
pensando que soy bugarrón.	thinking I am *bugarrón*
Pero están equivocadas	but they are totally wrong
porque más hembra que yo	more *hembra* than me
no encontrarán en la cama	in bed they'll never find.
Esto es una frustración,	This is such a frustration
tener este bello cuerpo,	to have this beautiful body,

pero te digo, mi hermana,	but I tell you, my sister,
que me cuesta mantenerlo.	it is hard to keep up.
El problema de este cuerpo	The problem with this body
es que me siguen las viejas	is that I'm followed by old ladies
y las locas, todas ellas,	and by queens, all of them,
y yo lo que estoy buscando	but what I'm really looking for
es una tranca bien regia.	Is a royal (huge) dick.
Casi desnuda, en la playa,	Half naked at the beach
paro el tráfico y me dicen	I stop traffic, and they tell me
"papi rico" y "mi machón"	"yummy daddy," "my big macho"
Y no saben que soy hembra	They can't tell I'm truly *hembra*
con este perro cuerpón.	with this amazing body of mine.
Pero no he perdido la ilusión	But I have not lost my fantasy
de que llegue Superman.	that Superman will arrive.
O irme a vivir a la selva	or go live in the jungle
y ser la mujer de Tarzán!	and become Tarzan's wife!

The poem speaks about the distress of a gay man whose masculine muscular body makes people, especially other gay men, believe that he is a real macho man (i.e., straight) or *bugarrón*, the word for heterosexual-identified men who sexually penetrate other men. In the poem, the gay man confesses that he really is an *hembra* (a real woman, feminine version of macho). The distress is caused by the fact that he is pursued by women and by *locas* (queens, homosexuals) rather than by real men, which is what he so deeply longs for.

The poem's logic is complex but clear: When homosexuality is defined in terms of gender, and homosexuals are not considered real men, it follows that homosexuals should not be sexually appealing to other homosexuals. The homosexual man, so the culture dictates, would desire another man, a real man, and therefore would not be interested in having sex with other homosexuals who are ultimately considered less than men.

When I first read the poem I had two different reactions. On one hand, I found the poem extremely humorous and provoking. The poem flaunts and cracks open what is supposedly the "big secret" of homosexuals: they may look masculine or even look like desirable real men—

"mi papi rico" (my sweet daddy), *"mi machón"* (my big macho man)—but they are truly women in men's bodies. Breaking the silence, and proudly flaunting society's ridiculing definition of homosexuality, the author expresses shamelessly his sexual desire for other men, his shameless longing for a huge dick. Somehow, there is humorous relief in such defiance of society's silence about homosexual desire.

On the other hand, I felt somewhat saddened by the fact that the familiar way to break the silence about homosexual desire, even in a gay magazine, is by taking a feminine identity. It is as if we can express our homosexual attraction openly only by talking not as men but as some type of woman or *hembra*, adopting the Latino culture's homophobic definition and point of view. I wonder if a similar lusty poem, written from one masculine man to another, would have appealed as much to the readership of *Perra!* I wouldn't be surprised if such a poem made many readers uncomfortable, stirring internalized homophobia. Or simply, from this particular perspective, it may not have made much sense to write such a poem for a gay audience. Not believing that homosexuals can be masculine, the reaction of many gay men could be: Why hide the *loca i*nside, when you are among understanding friends? Or as one of my research participants once commented about a masculine-looking, masculine-acting gay man, "Who does she think she is, she's a woman!"

Many times in the focus groups I conducted with non-acculturated, Spanish-speaking men, who in my sample were the ones less touched by gay liberation ideology, publicly coming out was referred to as *"se soltó la trenza"* (he undid his braid), meaning the achievement of a sense of freedom to be more effeminate, more womanlike. Others, when confronted with homophobic attitudes, mentioned that they would become more masculine in order to "pass" as straight men: "In my case I used a mustache to cover a bit."

Richard Parker, the noted ethnographer of Brazilian sexuality, once told me that in Brazil people would not blink an eye if they saw very effeminate men walking provocatively down the street, a sight not uncommon in many urban centers in Brazil. On the other hand, traffic would stop and riotlike conditions would develop if two masculine men with mustaches would dare to walk hand-in-hand down the street. The riots might be a comical exaggeration, but Richard's observation makes a lot of cultural sense from the perspective presented in this chapter.

I had similar mixed reactions when I saw the popular Cuban movie *Fresa y Chocolate* (Strawberry and Chocolate), which portrays an intelligent, handsome, sensitive, and simply adorable homosexual man befriending a somewhat naive, and unusually sensitive, straight man with whom he falls in love. The movie truly represents a great advance in Cuban society's tolerance towards homosexuality by breaking the silence about this otherwise taboo topic in such a positive way. (Remember that not too long ago, Cuban open homosexuals were put in jail, sent to work camps, or conveniently expatriated in the Mariel boat lift.) The fact that the gay man in the movie is portrayed as a likable, lovable character—even more deeply sensitive, cultured, and humane than his straight friend—is quite a feat in homosexual tolerance in comparison to other Latin American media, where homosexuals have been portrayed as depraved, immoral, low-world criminals or child molesters.

However, *Fresa y Chocolate*, directed by a self-identified heterosexual man, does not break free from the culture's gender definition of homosexuality. While the main character is still in man's clothes, his effeminate demeanor and non-masculine identification (symbolized by his choice of strawberry-flavored ice cream, rather than the more "masculine" chocolate) is made explicit time and again throughout the film. Not to mention the fact that the story is about a homosexual who sexually and romantically pursues a straight man. In fact, diverting from the original script written by a gay man, the heterosexual director added to the story a girlfriend with whom the straight man becomes sexually involved and falls in love. The addition of a girlfriend to the movie script by the heterosexual director was done apparently to make the straight character undoubtedly straight. As in Richard Parker's story about Brazilian men with mustaches, the possibility that a masculine man (our chocolate-identified character) could have homosexual feelings, especially nurturing and romantic feelings toward another man, is perhaps still too threatening for Cuban audiences to see. The girlfriend was a constant and convenient reminder that Mr. Chocolate was, indeed, no *Maricón*.

For many men, the path of liberation from oppressive gender ideologies includes being in touch with more "feminine" aspects of the self. No one can deny that the personal development toward human wholeness must include the integration of characteristics traditionally ascribed as masculine or feminine. Moreover, psychological research is very clear about the positive relationship between androgyny (defined as receiving test scores in the middle range between feminine and masculine extremes of gender identification) and psychological adjustment. However, I do not believe that the feminine identification seen in many Latino gay men is indeed a path toward wholeness or greater psychological adjustment. In fact, I see many of us deeply trapped in the oppressive gender ideologies that fuel homophobia in our communities. Rather than helping Latino homosexuals get in touch with feminine characteristics, the gender definition of homosexuality reinforces the macho ideal and its feminine counterpart, the *hembra*. For homosexuals, the outcome is not an increased social space for becoming whole, more integrated persons, but rather a caricature of an *hembra* in a macho body, as Tatiana's poem so well conveys.

The desperate attempts to prove our wounded masculinity or to experience the masculinity of our sexual partners keep us in the same macho-*hembra* dichotomous world and away from wholeness. Note, for example, that Tatiana's poem is filled with resigned self-deprecation, *"entre las piernas hay poco"* (there's little between the legs), while the most precious sexual object is *"una tranca bien regia"* (a royal huge dick). For the distressed gay man in the poem, only the realm of fantasy, rather than whole persons, can quench the thirst for the desired macho object: Superman or Tarzan might do.

Similarly, other homosexuals are put down and laughed at by homosexuals for not being men enough. It was not unusual for men in my research project to talk about other gay men as *"esas locas"* (those queens) in a true deprecatory way, or even worse "esas *locas pasivas*" (those passive queens), making it clear that the deprecation was in relation to taking "the woman's role" (*"el que hace de mujer"*) in sexual intercourse. And these self-deprecatory comments were made by men who openly admitted their homosexual interest in passive anal intercourse; in other words, they were putting down men like themselves. The character in Tatiana's poem, an admitted *"loca,"* mocks *"las locas"* that pursue him unsuspectedly. Moreover, such deprecatory mockery is not perceived as insulting to the gay men (the audience of *locas*) for whom the poem is written. This ever-present self-deprecation and deprecation of other homosexuals around the masculine ideal—though done mostly in the context of humor—in my opinion is a reflection of wounded self-esteem rather than a movement toward more integrative and liberating wholeness.

For many of us, it is true that if we want to be ourselves we need to do so by becoming softer and, from the point of view of the culture, more "effeminate." The path of liberation and wholeness does require giving up the need to prove our manhood and the compulsive need to conceal and repress the feminine in us. However, coming out has been defined not necessarily as a welcoming of the feminine, but rather as becoming more like the culturally defined *hembra*. It has become more a way to live the definition of homosexuality given to us by the culture, rather than a path of self-expression. The fact that coming out is defined as the freedom to be more *hembra* has bound us even further to a genderized, oppressive culture that seems to gender-type everything, even ice cream flavors. It is no surprise that homosexuality is gender-typed and sexual intercourse is clearly defined as active (masculine) or passive (feminine). Therefore, many men who sexually penetrate other men can do so in our culture without questioning their "heterosexual" (in their minds "masculine") identity.

Sexual Penetration: The Royal Road to Machohood

Our culture not only poses the challenge to prove masculinity but also provides specific means and avenues for doing so. The culture's definition of what constitutes manly or masculine behavior is acquired with particular poignancy by young Latino boys in the world of elementary school. Thus, a great deal of time and effort in the lives of Latino boys and youth is devoted to proving or showing off their masculinity through excellence in sports, through fights that establish hierarchies of power, through stories of defiant risk-taking activities, and, above all, through boasting sexual prowess.

Boys' stories about their sexual activity take on a particularly important role in establishing that they are indeed masculine macho men. It is not unusual for Latino youth to boast their sexual prowess through stories of sexual intercourse with older women who seduced them; stories of penetrating homosexual, effeminate boys who "let them do it" or older men who may "pay them to do it"; and, in rural areas, even stories of penetrating animals. Stories abound about fathers taking their sons early in their teenage years to be with prostitutes "so that they can finally become men." Needless to say, in this world of Latino male culture, sexual penetration becomes, to paraphrase Freud, the royal road to "machohood."

The strong connection between masculinity and penetration leads to a construction of sexuality as the favored locus to prove masculinity, an optimal place to restore the often wounded male ego. It is my belief that this construction is also present in men who enjoy passive intercourse. For them, the macho characteristics of the insertive partner and the potential strong and rough qualities of anal intercourse between two men play a major role in what is defined as pleasurable and erotic. The preoccupation of the insertive partner to maintain a long and strong erect penis for penetration, and the preoccupation of the receptive partner to be penetrated hard and heavy by a "real man," constitute two sides of the same coin: A sexuality designed to create, mend, and restore a sense of masculinity and macho ideal that are always under threat by the culture's demand to prove masculinity.

It is no surprise then that for many men in my qualitative study, especially the least acculturated, sex was defined narrowly and exclusively as penetration practices. Other sexual activity, such as deep kissing, caressing, and mutual masturbation were seen simply as preludes to the "real thing," penetration. Some men spoke about their sexual encounters as if orgasm and ejaculation were only possible in the context of penetration. Many feared that unless penetration occurred, their partners would be disappointed—that is, partners would perceive the encounter as bad sex or as having no sex at all. In fact, sexual activity without penetration was described often as "nothing really happened."

Impact on HIV Risk

The central thesis of this book is that important aspects of Latino culture—such as the link between machismo and homophobia in a gender definition of homosexuality—have been internalized by Latino gay men through our socialization and development. Such internalizations, in turn, have undermined our capacity for sexual self-regulation and become barriers to the practice of safer sex. In this section, therefore, I would like to explore the impact of machismo and homophobia on our sexuality and sexual behavior, especially those effects that are relevant to HIV prevention and the practice of safer sex.

This section is written with two underlying assumptions. The first assumption is that homophobia and machismo have deeply shaped the way we understand and perceive our own homosexuality, as well as how we sexually behave with other men. Thus, these barriers to safer sex are logical and meaningful through the cultural lens of how machismo and homophobia operate in our lives, as described in earlier sections of this chapter.

The second assumption is that barriers to safer sex will be more prevalent in those men who have been most deeply affected by the cultural link between machismo and homophobia. Latino gay men do vary in their internalization of the cultural factors, and also in their exposure and adherence to gay liberation ideologies. Fortunately, gender definitions of homosexuality are not present to the same degree in all of us, and the effects of machismo and homophobia are tempered by the increasing liberating awareness that men can sexually love other men without any detriment to their masculinity or masculine identity. Barriers to safer sex are stated, therefore, as variables that differ across individual members of the culture, rather than as fixed entities shared by us all.

Condoms and Erections

Because of the culture's connection between masculinity and penetrative practices, many men whom I interviewed expressed a great deal of concern about the negative effects of condoms on the sexual act. The main concern is that condoms, and their implicit connection to illness and death, would make them lose their erection.

> Sometimes if I think too much about it I might lose my erection. Because sex isn't enjoyable anymore 'cuz you are thinking about disease, disease, disease, you know.

Moreover, the loss of erection is perceived as a source of great embarrassment by the insertive partner, yet another failure at masculinity. The loss of an erection is apparently equated with the collapse of the macho façade that reveals the true *loca pasiva* inside, giving precisely the wrong message to the demanding, now disappointed, receptive partner: "And he kept on saying, why can't you get it hard? why can't you get it hard?"

The concern with maintaining erections at all cost does not allow the time needed for the gradual familiarization with and erotization of condoms.

Impact on Non-Penetrative Practices

Mutuality and nurturance in sexual behavior is often interpreted as non-masculine, taking away the erotic charge for those men who have accepted the gender definition of homosexuality. For men who enjoy their masculinity and thus have trouble identifying themselves as homosexual, caressing, kissing, and passive oral sex to other men is out of the question. Many acculturated men complained a lot about those non-acculturated Latino macho guys, who do not consider themselves gay and who defend their masculinity by not doing "gay things" in homosexual acts. These heterosexual-identified men who have sex with men, in fact, define their manhood by what they do and not do in bed with another guy. Moreover, denial of gay identification in homosexual activity goes hand-in-hand with a denial of HIV risk:

> I know there's a lot of straight "macho" Latin guys that think, "Oh, you're just sucking my dick or I'm gonna fuck you and I have a wife or I have a girlfriend so it really doesn't mean that I'm gay and we can have unsafe sex because I only have sex with girls" and, you know. That whole sort of thinking that goes along with other Latin men.

For those men who share the gender-definition of homosexuality, anything other than actively fucking another man is considered non-masculine and a threat to the heterosexual, macho identity. In turn, self-identified homosexuals who have adopted the feminine *loca* identity may be sexually turned-off by attempts at sexual mutuality. As one of the men in the study said, "If he touches my dick, I am not interested anymore." The comment implied that any attempt at mutuality would mean that the sexual partner was also an effeminate loca and therefore not sexually appealing to the study subject, who was interested only in masculine "real" men.

It is clear that the construction of sexuality as a place to create and prove masculinity poses some major challenges and obstacles for the enactment of safer sex intentions. The exclusive focus on penetration does not allow Latino gay men to explore and develop a repertoire of non-penetrative safer sex practices that can be enjoyed as true expressions of sexual desire. The machismo message given by the culture does not allow much space for the kind of caring and nurturing that is needed for the negotiation of safer sex between sexual partners.

Substance Abuse and Anonymous Sex

Homosexual activity in the context of machismo and homophobia messages is loaded with a deep anxiety that what is happening is disgusting and forbidden. It is no surprise that sex between gay men often occurs anonymously, with strangers in strange places, with no communication, and under the influence of drugs and alcohol, or both.

A large number of men in the study reported that they were intoxicated while looking for sexual partners as well as during homosexual encounters. Some of them talked about needing alcohol and drugs to give them the "courage" to meet and approach other men for sex. Others talked about using substances to help them engage in practices that they wanted to do but felt very uneasy about, especially anal intercourse. Men told stories about using alcohol and drugs, especially before coming out to themselves and others, as a justification for "not remembering" things they wanted to do or had done, but were too embarrassed to admit. For example, being under the influence of substances was the only possible way to have sex between friends who were sexually attracted to one another but who had never discussed or revealed their homosexuality to each other; being under the influence allowed the friends to make believe that they did not remember so at a later date they could face one another without shame.

For men who want to be sexually penetrated, but for whom playing the passive role in anal intercourse creates masculinity conflicts, drugs and alcohol have become the facilitating factor. Recent increases in the use of methamphetamines ("crystal" or "speed") among gay men have been also observed among Latinos as a way to deal with ambivalent feelings regarding anal intercourse. For some, the drug facilitates taking the passive role: "It [crystal] makes me an eager bottom." Many men welcomed drug intoxication as a true oasis of relief from the masculinity anxiety brought about by homosexual sex. In the words of a 31-year-old Latino gay man, for whom the crystal methamphetamine (speed) intoxication allowed him to enjoy the sense of (gender-role-free) mutuality he craved with his lover:

> I felt more like the top in the relationship, in that I kind of controlled things more. Again, it was like my space and I brought him into it. You know, I was more in charge of like paying bills and things like that. So I felt like more of the—I don't want to say masculine and feminine because, you know, I don't find these roles like, you know, okay, that's what that means. But I was more like the husband in the situation and just sexually I was more aggressive. And so, I mean, I think that the speed just turned everything kind of like really topsy-turvy where we were just kind of like, you know, not been thinking about roles any more, just kind of what felt good.

For other men, for whom keeping erections is a problem, stimulant drugs was the only way to maintain their erection in the midst of anxiety-provoking situations.

In one of the in-depth interviews conducted by the San Francisco AIDS Foundation, Antonio (fictitious name)—a 31-year-old, HIV-positive, Latino gay man—told the interviewer about a risky sexual encounter where neither he nor his partner used a condom. The two men met through one of San Francisco's (900#) sex phone lines; the service connects via phone lines men who are interested in meeting other men for sex and who call the service for that purpose. I would like to cite long excerpts from this narrative because the sexual episode described involved many of the cultural factors and barriers to safer sex discussed in this section. Both partners, one gay-identified Latino (Antonio) and a presumably straight man of Italian descent, attempted to construct the sexual situation in terms of an exchange between two "straight" men, ensuring that the sexual event is truly an experience of masculinity. Furthermore, the event occurred in secrecy, as a hidden encounter, behind closed doors, so that the "straight roommates" would not find out what was going on. Both men were intoxicated with drugs and alcohol, including crystal. In fact, Antonio makes the attribution that it is crystal that has allowed him to carry out all this forbidden activity. Early on in the interview, he had talked about being a top in the majority of sexual situations. However, for this episode, he had taken crystal and, because impotence can be one of the paradoxical effects of methamphetamine use, commonly known as "crystal dick," the drug made him lose his erection and made him "an eager bottom."

Antonio: ... I met this guy on the phone line, he was an Italian guy ... you know he's very "macho" and straight and, you know, has a girlfriend, and no one would ever know that he was doing something like this but he felt like doing it tonight, because he had been partying too. He had been doing "coke" the night before with his friends. And—

Interviewer: And you were feeling?

A: Like I wanted to have sex.

I: OK. Specifically, you wanted to fuck?

A: Yeah. I think that's what the drug does to, at least it does to me. It just puts you in that whole mind set of like, I have to go out and find something.

I: Something meaning a ... sex?

A: Sex!

I: A sexual partner.

A: Right.

I: OK. So you talked to him on the phone?

A: Yeah.

I: Made the arrangements?

A: Right. Went over to his place.

I: In [name of a "straight" neighborhood in San Francisco]?

A: Yes! Um, he was pretty partied-out. So we smoked some "pot" when we got there and had a couple beers. Had we just had the pot and the beers I could handle that because I've done that a lot.

I: You mean handle in terms of what's gonna happen next with sex?

A: Right. What's gonna happen with sex. I'm very in control but I don't think I am when I've been doing crystal. So, um, he was pretty, he, I don't know, he tried to be insistent at one point on having safe sex but then he changed his mind like really quickly.

I: Were you still dressed when he was being insistent? Do you remember?

A: Oh. Well, let me go back. So we got there, okay. We talked for a while and he had some porno on the TV and we had to be really quiet because he had straight roommates coming in and out and they had no idea that this was goin' on in his bedroom, so we never left the bedroom.

I: So you walked into the apartment and went right to his room?

A: Right.

I: And none of his roommates knew that he had sex with men?

A: Supposedly. I mean I heard the front door slamming and pots in the kitchen. I tried to ask him some questions about his roommates but he wouldn't answer me. Uh, he was pretty secretive.

I: So that was okay though?

A: Yeah. For the way I was feeling at that time, yeah. Had I been a little more clearer thinking, I think I probably wouldn't have gone over there. But he said, you know, do you wanna come over, we'll keep partying and I was like already in a party mood so I said, "OK." And I got there, he was very attractive, very, I would never thought if I saw him on the street, you know, that he would do something like this. Whatever.

I: You mean the partying part or the . . .

A: Uh.

I: . . . the keeping you in his bedroom while his roommates are running around, part or . . . ?

A: Having sex with a guy.

I: I can't tell who has sex with guys or with gals on the street.

A: I know, you know, it's like supposedly gay men have this "gay-dar" and they can tell who's gay and who's not, and I'm pretty much on the dot all the time as to who's gay and who's not, and who would maybe fool around if you convinced him and who wouldn't. And I just woulda never thought looking at this guy. He looked like very, like he coulda been a butcher or a cook in like an Italian restaurant. Sort of burly, hairy, short, stocky, muscular, I could see him with like a wife and kids. Who knows. So I think he called a friend of his when I got there, to bring over some more coke. And in the meantime we smoked some pot, had a beer, slowly disrobed 'til we were naked in bed. His friend got there and I think I did . . . yeah, some coke. Yeah, after being on crystal, which was . . .

I: Did his friend see you?

A: No. He met him at the door. And, um, so he wanted to be fucked too, which I thought was very peculiar. I mean, I don't know. I, and

I tried for a while but I couldn't get an erection because of the crystal.

I: Did he know you had taken crystal?

A: Yeah, I told him.

I: Does he know, since he's not part of the community, does he know things like what "crystal dick" is?

A: He didn't. Yeah. I was kind of amazed, I guess. Because he kept on saying, "Why can't you get it hard? Why can't you get it hard?" And I was like, "I told you because this drug affects me this way that I did last night." So he goes well, "Just relax, just relax and don't think about it and it'll happen." So, whatever, so, you know. So then he said, "Well, why don't I fuck you?" So um, so we started talkin' about using a condom and then I don't know exactly how it happened but we didn't.

I: So you're already in bed, you already had your clothes off? Did you take each other's clothes off each other or . . .

A: No. There wasn't any sort of sensual, intimate . . .

I: No foreplay?

A: No. It was kind of sort of almost like a raunchy aspect of it.

I: Did you think he was attractive?

A: Yeah.

I: So you talked about using a condom but then it didn't happen?

A: Well actually what happened was I think at one point, he put one on and he was having problems keeping an erection himself, so then he took it off and we continued.

I: So he just simply took the condom off? Did he masturbate, anything like that?

A: Uh, yeah, we masturbated for quite a while by just watching porno, and I was oral with him, he wasn't oral with me, he didn't want to do that. He didn't want to kiss, he didn't want to suck my dick. So I was doing all the work.

I: Why didn't he wanna do those things, do you think?

A: Because maybe that meant to him that he was gay. If he didn't kiss you and he didn't suck your dick if you just sucked his dick and he fucked you, then he's not gay. But then he also wanted to be fucked, which I thought was kinda weird but he said it was because, and this was a clinical problem for him, that his brother had sex with him growing up. So maybe he's going through this whole incest thing. I don't know.

I: So he volunteered up that information . . .

A: Yeah.

I: . . . about himself but he didn't volunteer . . .

A: Yeah, and the sick . . .

I: . . . a lotta other . . .

A: Well, the sick thing about it was that he wanted, he wanted me to even make up stories that we were having sex, like acting like I was his brother having sex with him. I mean it was kind of unsettling.

I: For you?

S: Yeah. But I didn't . . .

I: What did it feel like?

S: Uh, feeling like this was really weird. It was just like one a' those weird experiences.

I: Did it feel dangerous?

S: Yeah, it did.

I: How dangerous? Because we've used the word danger in relationship to other things. How did it feel dangerous?

S: Um, it didn't feel dangerous in the aspect that I thought that he would get violent with me. It got dangerous in the fact that I felt somehow I was gonna get an erection. He was gonna convince me to have sex with him without a condom and I was gonna' come inside him which I did not wanna do.

I: Did you talk about HIV at all when you were with him?

S: No.

I: He never mentioned it? So did you talk about condom usage as safe sex or just using one?

S: We didn't even talk about it, he just got up and went over and got one.

I: Ah! OK. Because it wasn't . . .

S: And said something like, "We should be using one of these," or something like that.

I: So the word HIV didn't come up?

S: No.

I: Did he ask you about your serostatus?

S: No.

I: Did he see you as gay?

S: Um, you know, that's the funny thing, not really. I mean he asked me a coupla questions. And I said "I mainly have sex with men and it's been ages since I had sex with a woman." And uh, he said, "Wow! You don't seem to be gay to me." Which I think I can be pretty gay, you know. So whatever that is. I don't know if it was just because he was partying and he was flying high. But he seemed to wanna make me feel like you're not gay you're just a straight buddy a' mine and we're gonna play, sorta thing.

I: So it sounds like you understood. And did you understand this in the moment or did you understand it later, that he had a big fantasy thing going on?

S: While it was happening I was like, even though I was high, I was like, I think he's fulfilling a fantasy right now and I'm being part of it.

I: Um hm. OK. So did he come inside of you?

S: Yes.

I: Um hm. How'd you feel about it?

S: Really stupid! I mean, it felt good but, you know, have you ever done something and know you're doing something wrong and you should not be doing it, and you should stop yourself but you continue to do it?

In this amazing narrative we see the intertwining of a masculinity fantasy with perhaps what could be the compulsive repetition of a sexual abuse experience, all of it embedded in the stupor of heavy drug use, allowing men to do what they would otherwise be too anxious to do without the use of substances. The end result is, of course, a highly risky episode from the perspective of HIV transmission. Even though our Latino respondent blames crystal, the narrative does conclude with a pervasive feeling of helplessness, contributing to a perception of low sexual control that is familiar to many other Latinos for reasons other than drugs.

Perceptions of Sexual Control

A consistent theme throughout the interviews I conducted was the perception that Latino men have little control of their sexuality. The belief is that Latino men are supposed to experience intense feelings, urges, and sensations that cannot or should not be controlled. For example, the men I interviewed often used the notion of being "passionate" as a justification for unprotected intercourse. Passionate, however, refers not only to the intensity of the feelings and sensations experienced, but also to the surrender of inhibitions, the surrender of self-control and regulation in the presence of intense sexual feelings. In other words, passionate meant that intense "hot" feelings took precedence over and were not mediated by "cold" decision-making or thinking processes that could temper the intensity of the experience. I should add that this self-perception of intense, passionate, and personal surrender to the dictates of sexual arousal is often reinforced when projected on Latino gay men by members of the mainstream gay culture in a stereotypical fashion.

The perception of low sexual control is, I believe, also strongly connected to the machismo values of the Latino culture. The idea is that men's sexual urges are felt delightfully but painfully strong and thus require immediate release; men's sexual urges cannot be ignored, postponed, or ultimately controlled. Accordingly, males are expected to have multiple casual partners and their sexual activity is expected to occur more often as a response to strong, biologically based impulses rather than as an expression of love and affection in the context of interpersonal relationships. Females, in contrast, are expected to control and not even feel their sexual desires; if their sexual desires or behavior do not occur in the context of relationships then they are considered immoral, depraved, or prostitutes. In the words of a Latino gay man I interviewed:

> I was very close to my father's mother. She would always tell us about all the women my father slept with and it was something everybody knew and we had to accept it.... I remember she would say "this is your father's other woman, he is just sleeping with her, but that's OK." My grandmother would also tell me that was OK. My uncle would say things like I love your aunt but you know its OK to have another woman.... I have a very big problem with that and it really hurt me and it always really hurt me that my father would do that to my mother but no I guess its OK and then I started looking at the women my father was sleeping with like sluts, whores because they're doing that knowing that he was married. My grandmother was the type of woman that

would degrade women that cheated on their husbands but on the other hand it was OK for my father to cheat. Looking back I think that was the thing about machismo that bothered me the most about it.

In support of a self-perception of low sexual control, the men interviewed shared the belief that regulatory control of sexual behavior is not possible at times of high sexual arousal; the higher the arousal, the less control possible. This perception was epitomized by the well-known phrase, *"Cuando la de abajo se calienta, la de arriba no piensa,"* literally translated as, "When the one below gets hot, the one on top can't think." the "one" refers to "head," of which males have two: the head of the penis (below), and the head that contains the thinking brain (on top). The belief is that sexual arousal interferes with or inhibits thinking processes, as if sexual arousal and rational decision-making processes cannot happen simultaneously within the person. It is not surprising that many men used this perception or colorful phrase as a way to justify instances of unprotected sex in what they believed was a socially accepted pattern of Latino male behavior:

> You know, when you're in the heat of passion, you're not going to be concerned with wearing a rubber, you are just going to go for it at that point, but I think a lot of people aren't going to stop and say, "now I have to put on a rubber.". . . Part of that is the natural passion that's going on . . .

Coda: The National Context

In October 1995, the Public Media Center in San Francisco produced an in-depth (and in my opinion), brilliant analysis of the impact of homophobia on the spread of HIV and AIDS in the U.S. The report, entitled "The impact of homophobia and other social biases on AIDS," describes how the definition of AIDS as a gay disease, and the linkage between AIDS and gay issues in the mind of the general public, has produced what is perhaps the major barrier—AIDS-Related Stigma—against a focused, coherent, and effective national effort to fight this devastating disease. The report forcefully concludes that

> the unaddressed issue of homophobia remains the unseen cause of the spread of AIDS-Related Stigma within U.S. society. We believe that

until the issue of homophobia is properly and adequately addressed in America, our nation is unlikely to generate an objective, focused response to the epidemic of HIV and AIDS. (PMC, 1995, p. 5)

In seemingly parallel universes, approximately one month before the 1996 presidential elections, our country was bombarded with a distressing homophobic discourse. President Bill Clinton signed the ban on homosexual marriages and the California legislature held hearings on Governor Wilson's proposal to restrict adoptions to heterosexual parents.

The news is not good. Keeping with the highly politicized homophobic debates, the *San Francisco Chronicle* recently published the results of the 1991 General Social Survey, periodically conducted by the National Opinion Research Center at the University of Chicago. The title of the article "Public opinion of homosexuals stays negative," is somewhat deceiving, because the article in truth reports a slight worsening of public opinion regarding homosexuality. The article states:

According to the 1977 General Social Survey, the country's most-watched barometer of social trends and attitudes, 67 percent of those questioned said that sex between two adults of the same sex was "always wrong." In the 1991 survey, 71 percent said gay sex was always wrong.

Similarly, perhaps in more subtle ways, the nation's machismo discourse is very much alive. The words of praise for Scott O'Grady, the Air Force captain who survived six days behind enemy lines after being shot by Serbian rebel forces, were definitely about his masculinity: "This is a tough *hombre* we are talking about—Adm. L. Smith" (*S.F. Chronicle*, June 9, 1995). Setting aside the provocative fact that Admiral Leighton Smith used the Spanish word for man (*hombre*) when talking about the manhood of an Irish American, it is important to note that both the military and the press constructed the heroic events in terms of the culture's masculine ideal.

About the same time, published in 1995, Michael Kimmel's insightful analysis of masculinity links the resurgence of social prejudices in our country to the often wounded male ego of American men. In the words of the book's reviewer:

The pattern recurs throughout American history. Men feel their power
waning on account of an economic downturn or, so they believe, on
account of the gains of previously subordinated groups. Feeling threatened as men, they react defensively. Some seek new avenues to prove
their manhood: Westward Ho!, making war, building stronger bodies,
escape into imaginary worlds peopled by superheroes, etc. . . . Then, failing these pursuits, they project the menace onto classes of people over
whom they still wield some power, be these people of color, immigrants,
women or gays. (Kupers, 1995, p. 19)

Considering the issues raised in this chapter, and reflecting on the
nation's sociopolitical discourse as we approach the second millennium,
I am tempted to re-write the conclusion of the Public Media Center
report as follows: "Until the issue(s) of homophobia (and machismo)
is(are) properly and adequately addressed in America . . ."

5.

Family Loyalty
and Sexual Silence

Splitting Off Sexuality

Interviewer: For you, what is the most difficult thing about being a Latino gay man?

Respondent: Hurting my family.

In both group and individual interviews, the topic of "family" was introduced rather early and spontaneously by Latino gay men, in response to introductory questions about the difficulties encountered in their lives. During the interviews, I witnessed abundant stories of family rejection, including the often-heard, cruel, parental saying, *"Mi hijo, mejor muerto que maricón"* (My son, better dead than a faggot). Stories of family rejection, however, were typically told compassionately, at times apologetically, emphasizing not the hurt of the rejected son but rather the pain caused by bringing shame and dishonor to those they loved the most.

I also witnessed stories of family acceptance and support. Some of the men I interviewed experienced their family as a haven of security, as an "inside world" that served as a refuge from a hostile and cruel machista, homophobic world. In the words of a 42-year-old man, originally from Mexico City:

Being a gay male, of course, I was target to a lot of jokes and things. So I guess what helped me kind of continue growing was just kind of finding refuge in my own family because being in contact with the outside world, it always kind of meant teasing or mocking, things like that.

However, with further inquiry, stories about family support were mostly stories of tolerance and non-abuse rather than of true acceptance. In most cases, tolerance was achieved only at the price of silence about their homosexuality. The interview with the man from Mexico City quoted above continued as follows:

I feel that I probably could take the jokes or whatever about being pointed as a, you know, little gay boy, but the thing that was very difficult was when I felt very vulnerable that I would be with my family and they would whistle at me or some kind of thing that would expose me to my own family. . . . [Nowadays], with the family, we don't talk about it, even though it's very understood. There is absolutely no doubt in my mind that they all know about my life, but we don't talk about it. And it's basically with my family that I'm more reserved but with friends . . . my friends, they all know and I can be very open about it.

Interviewer: Tell me a little more about the sort of understanding with your family. What are the indicators that they know and they understand?

Respondent: The indicators are that I think I was a very effeminate little boy and I don't ever remember my family putting me down for just being who I was, and as I developed into adolescence I think I stopped being effeminate but I was more in touch with my own desires and sexuality. And when I was 16 years old, I started my gay life and I was never ashamed or embarrassed to bring my gay friends home and sometimes they were pretty obvious. So to me the indicators were like my family sees me surrounded by these very unusual type people and yet they don't put it down or anything. They just kind of allow it to happen and me be myself.

I: But it's never been openly discussed?

R: It's never been openly discussed.

In the context of focus-group discussions, it was fascinating to observe the reaction of group members to a participant's detailed description of family rejection. While most men laughed and joked at some of the stories of faggot mocking and teasing by their peers, stories of family rejection brought a disturbing silence to the group. The majority of men listened very attentively, nodding silently, some with tears in their eyes, as if saying "you are not alone." In fact, in commenting about the group experience at the end of focus-group sessions, many men commented upon how important, and what a relief, it had been for them to hear how other men had similar family stories.

Other men would counteract and talk about how their families were different, and how much their families had accepted them. In most cases, however, the "acceptance" stories would reconfirm the price of silence.

Me apoyan . . . sospecho que saben que soy gay, pues mi familia no es estúpida, pero nunca han hablado de eso. (They support me . . . I suspect that they know that I'm gay, because my family is not stupid, but they've never talked about it.)

A handful of men were able to tell stories of family acceptance, achieved mostly through a courageous and militant breaking of the homosexual silence. In these cases, men confronted their families, lovingly but firmly, about who their "true" son was. Acceptance came when the family, courageously and against all kinds of cultural prejudice, met their children's challenge. These families valued a strong participation and inclusion in their son's life more than *"el qué dirán"* (what others would say). With time, these families would become more and more involved with their children's lives, including their boyfriends and lovers, their gay activism, and, in some cases, their HIV disease.

This handful of cases reporting family acceptance typically contained militant, activist men who were very articulate about their experiences of oppression, and who were committed to stop such oppression for themselves and their communities. These men were well aware of the damaging effects of silence in their lives and, in the context of the focus groups, would argue that our fears about openly telling our parents are often unfounded: "I thought my father was going to die of a heart attack if I told him, but he didn't." As Victor, one of the most articulate participants in the earliest stages of my research, who recently and painfully died of AIDS before his 30th birthday, told me: *"El gran problema del problema es no hablar del problema"* (The big problem of the problem is not talking about the problem).

My qualitative research has yielded four clear facts about Latino gay men's relationships to their families. First, there is an immense sense of respect, affiliation, and loyalty to family of origin, even in the face of difficult experiences of rejection and disdain. Family loyalty is manifested mostly by taking the family's point of view in painful and potentially shameful situations. Second, very few men have experienced "true" family support, that is, support that would include an overt and sincere welcome and acceptance of their children's homosexuality. Family support, when reported, was mostly experienced as tolerance, parental resignation, or the absence of overt mocking and abuse. Even in the stories about the most supportive families, I never heard of a family who would give a proud and enthusiastic welcome to their son's homosexual orientation. Third, the majority of men expressed that family members knew about their being gay, even though they never talked about it. In fact, for the overwhelming majority of men, silence about their sexuality was the only way to experience family (and societal) "support." For many, breaking the silence, even in families who already knew, was the beginning of serious family conflict that led to disruption of family ties, including migration or expatriation. Fourth, it became crystal clear that the relationship to family of origin is extremely central to Latino gay men's lives, regardless of age, and that this relationship has a profound impact on their current sexual lives and homosexual relationships.

Familism

It is a well-known and documented fact that Latinos have an enormous regard and place a very high value on family life and the interpersonal relations among family members. This central value of Latino culture has been termed "familism" by researchers in the field.

According to Marín and Marín (1991), familism is "a cultural value that involves individuals' strong identification with and attachment to their nuclear and extended families, and strong feelings of loyalty, reciprocity, and solidarity among members of the same family" (p. 13). The importance of family relations and the actual close involvement of families in the lives and affairs of the individual members is not considered a temporary situation of youth, but rather a life-long commitment that connects individuals, even after marriage, to a relatively large and supportive social network of caring and concerned human beings.

Interestingly, familism values among Latinos, especially high levels of perceived family support, are very resistant to change in response to acculturation into the U.S. mainstream culture. Sabogal et al. (1987), in a study of 452 Hispanics and 227 non-Hispanic Whites, examined ethnic group and acculturation differences on a scale of familism. The scale measured three different dimensions: familial obligations, family support, and family as social referent. The study revealed no significant differences in familismo values among the three groups of Hispanics studied: Mexican, Central, and Cuban Americans. The authors thus concluded that familism is "a core characteristic in the Hispanic culture" (p. 397). Even though there were some declines in familism values due to increasing acculturation for both dimensions of "familial obligations" and "family as referent," the "perceived level of family support" remained unchanged with increased acculturation. Moreover, on all three dimensions of familism, Hispanics scored significantly higher than their non-Hispanic White counterparts. The study did not report respondents' sexual orientation or sexual self-identification (nor is there evidence that these were assessed); however, it can be assumed from the reported sampling strategies that the respondents were, in their overwhelming majority, heterosexual men and women (approximately 60% of the sample was female).

Latinos are aware and proud of this shared familism cultural value and use it to define themselves in contrast to "Anglos" (the name most commonly used by my research participants in reference to non-Hispanic Whites). For example, when Latinos talk about themselves in comparison to the Anglo mainstream culture—as I witnessed in many of the research interviews—they often refer to the distance and coldness of relations among Anglo family members and about their puzzlement at how Anglos "leave their families behind when they turn 18" or how "even some of them talk bad about their parents."

It is important to note that in Latin American cultures, as explained by Carballo-Diéguez (1989), the concept of family

> encompasses more than the immediate family. Grandparents are considered an integral and important part of the family. . . . Aunts, uncles, their children, and even more distant relatives are also considered part of what

is known as the "extended family." Then there are the compadres and comadres, people very close to the family, because they are the godparents of a child, because they come from the same hometown, or simply because they are good old friends. (p. 28)

Membership in such an extensive and resourceful social network provides individuals with a sense of security and social connectedness that protects them from both economic hardship and social isolation or loneliness. Marín and Marín (1991) note that familism provides a natural support system that protects individuals from both physical and emotional stress. For Latinos in the U.S., social support within the family system constitutes one of the most important protective factors against the health risks posed by poverty and minority status (García-Coll, 1990).

Familism in Latino Gay Men

For homosexuals, on the other hand, familism values can represent something other than an asset when families perceive their children's homosexuality as sinful, immoral, and shameful. The strong ties within Latino families, and the major role that families play in the care and support of Latino individuals, can become (and usually is) a major source of conflict and tension for homosexuals (Ceballos-Capitaine et al., 1990). As I argued at the beginning of this chapter, social support within homophobic families can be achieved only at the expense of self-expression and openness about the individual member's homosexuality; acceptance by and social connectedness to the family are achieved and maintained only at the price of silence. The conflict is experienced as a painful choice within a no-win situation, a choice between self-expression and family love.

Familism values, as strong in Latino homosexuals as in any other members of the Latino culture, prevent homosexuals from denouncing the family's homophobia and demanding acceptance. Instead, for the sake of psychological connectedness and identification with the family, homophobia tends to become internalized in a self-punitive way. I believe that this is why in my interviews Latino gay men seldom complained about their parents' and family members' rejection. Instead, taking the point of view of the family, they talked about how difficult it is to live with the fact that their homosexuality hurts their parents.

> My parents have worked very hard, they have lived a very hard life, sacrificing themselves for their children, and now they have to deal with this shame . . . it is a very serious blow to them.

The majority of men interviewed spoke with great sadness about the pain that their homosexuality has caused their family. They seldom expressed anger at the families for the pain that they themselves have experienced due to their families' homophobic rejection. In some cases, family members with whom the men had spoken openly about their homosexuality counseled them to remain silent with other family members in order "not to hurt" more people in the family.

> *Mi tia me dijo, para qué herir y lastimar a otros [familiares]? Para qué preocuparlos?* (My aunt told me, Why wound and cause hurt in others [family members]? Why cause them worry?)

My hypothesis and tentative conclusion is that the most important expression and manifestation of familism values among homosexuals is precisely keeping silent about their homosexuality. Rather than a protective value, the strong loyalty to family—and its expression in sexual silence—has an enormous and detrimental impact on the well-being, sexual behavior, and ultimately HIV risk of Latino homosexuals.

Some Consequences of Familism for Gay Men

There are some serious consequences, with direct relevance to HIV risk, of having such a strong bond to homophobic families. For one, personal and social identification as a homosexual—that is, coming out to yourself and to others—becomes extremely difficult. Since closeted and hidden lives do not allow individuals to deal effectively with and recover from their own internalized homophobia, issues of low self-esteem and personal shame about homosexual desire are abundant among Latino gay men. Homosexual feelings are experienced with some resentment because these feelings are recognized as the source of disruption and estrangement from the highly valued and potentially protective family support system.

> *[Mi madre] me enseñó muchas cosas muy religiosas y me dirigió la mente por el camino heterosexual. . . . Cuando yo empecé a sentir mis relaciones, después que pasé mi pubertad, tuve un complejo de inferioridad increíble. Yo odiaba mi personalidad, deseaba no haber nacido, traté dos veces de quitarme la vida. Y yo culpaba a Dios. Yo pedía "que me quites esto," quería que me gustaran las muchachas.* ([My mother] taught me a lot of religious things and directed my mind toward the heterosexual path. When I started to [feel my sexual relations], after I went through puberty, I had a great inferiority complex. I hated my personality, I wished I hadn't been born, and I attempted suicide twice. I blamed God. I prayed "please take [homosexual feelings] away," I wanted to like girls.)

Because coming out to the family involves the risk of hurting or losing them, it happens only partially, only with selected people, and often in selected places that have no direct connection to or contact with the family.

> *Y ya me andaba casando, y me dí cuenta que no iba a ser feliz y tuve mis aventuras afuera, todo lo que tenía que hacer, muy lejos de mi casa, lejos de mi familia, a escondidas, lejos de mis amigos.* (I was ready to get married and then I realized that I wasn't going to be happy, and I had my adventures [homosexual encounters] outside, all I had to do I did far away from home, hidden, far away from my friends.)

For those individuals who remain in close connection to their families, identification with and participation in family life requires that their sexual lives, their sexual partners or lovers, and their gay friends be excluded from the social, affective network of family membership. Thus, a second consequence of relating to homophobic families is a *forced separation between individuals' sexuality and their social, affective life.* It is no surprise that for Latino gay men who try to keep a strong and active connection to family life, sex and relationships become progressively disconnected, sexual behavior is pushed toward the context of anonymous, hidden encounters and out of the affective, social domain. Many of these men participate in family reunions, family dinners, family holiday events, at times bringing "girlfriends" to those events in order to please (or not hurt) their parents and cover up their homosexuality. Frequently, right after the family events, right after taking their girlfriends home and kissing them goodnight, these men go to parks, truck stops, or public restrooms to have sex with other men, typically with strangers and in strange hidden places. Sexuality is thus constructed as the domain of the secret and the forbidden, mentally and functionally disconnected from affective and social relationships.

Some homosexual men, well aware of their strong homosexual desires and orientation, get married in order to participate more fully and more comfortably in the social life of their extended family. Through marriage they can partake of the immense protective benefits and social support of family life. These men's sexual release and fulfillment can only happen "on the side," either by having secret lovers whom they meet for quick sexual encounters or by having anonymous sex. It seems clear that the high frequency of bisexual behavior found among Latinos is due not only to the fact that heterosexual men are allowed to find sexual release with other men but also to the large number of truly (but secretly) homosexually identified men who have chosen married life as a way to solve the homophobic family dilemma. The sense of losing family life as a natural consequence of accepting and living one's homosexuality is so strong that even gay-identified Latino men who live openly within the gay community often talk about their frustrated dreams of getting married and having children not only to create their own families but also as a way to reconnect with their own extended families.

The late Cuban writer Reynaldo Arenas, in his autobiography *Before the Night Falls*, documented with both passion and artistry the high frequency of homosexual activity in Castro's Cuba, all of it of course "underground," creating a sexuality forcibly hidden on account of family values.

> Men would go to the beach with their wives and sit on the sand to relax; but sometimes they would go to the changing booths, have erotic adventures with other young men, and then return to their wives. I remember a particularly good-looking man playing with his son and wife in the sand. He would lie down, lift his legs, and I could see his beautiful testicles. I watched him playing with his son for a long time, lifting his legs

and showing me his testicles. Finally he went to the changing-booth building, took a shower, and went up to get dressed. I followed him; I think I asked him for a cigarette or a match, and he invited me in. For five minutes he was unfaithful to his wife in the most astonishing ways. Later I saw him again with his wife on his arm and his son, a beautiful family picture. (p. 100)

Arenas himself, a deeply committed homosexual, open to himself and many others in Cuba, struggled with anguish about his family loyalty. One obvious solution, of course, was to take the same path as his changing-booth partner, something his mother wanted him to do, but something he really could not get himself to do. Like many of my research participants, Arenas wrote the story from the point of view of his mother's pain, expressing his pain only for hurting his mother so badly, and ultimately blaming himself for his mother's loneliness.

Before getting to my mother's house, I would always think of her on the porch or even on the street, sweeping. . . . Perhaps with that broom she tried to sweep all the horrors, all the loneliness, all the misery that had accompanied her all her life, and me, her only son, now a homosexual in disgrace and persecuted as a writer. . . . My mother's nightmare was that I would end up in jail. Every time I visited her in Oriente she asked me to get married. Her request was so sad and so absurd. I would finally let her persuade me. Why not give that woman, who had known so few joys in life, one last pleasure? She wanted me to have a son and to bring him to her so her old age would not be so lonely. And I would return to Havana sadder than when I left. (pp. 142–43)

The disconnection between sexuality and affective life, experienced many times as loneliness and longing for a romantic relationship, push many Latino gay men toward anonymous encounters. Many report that, in these hidden encounters, they act in ways they really don't want to act. In those situations, they feel little possibility of control, at times watching themselves as if they were watching someone else. This subjective experience of psychological dissociation was experienced as a "disembodied trance" by Jorge (fictitious name), a 30-year-old Latino gay man, in the context of an unprotected sexual encounter in a cruising park. The experience was prompted by deep feelings of loneliness brought by a frustrated attempt at a romantic relationship with "R."

> I was down about "R" and I was feeling lonely. And from there I decided to go home but instead I ended up going out cruising to a park. I went up there quickly and found someone who seemed interested. He performed oral sex on me and then he turned around and dropped his pants and I started to fuck him. I remember saying something about a condom, neither of us had one but we went ahead and did it anyways. We did that for not very long, maybe like a minute, and then he wanted to go somewhere else to continue. So we went somewhere else, we continued and I pulled out just as I was about to come. And then he turned around and to my surprise he started going down on me again after I had just fucked him without a condom and then I came.
>
> I was uh, very shocked immediately afterwards. And I was particularly like frightened that he had, after I had been fucking him, turned around and gone down on me again. I kept thinking about that and I was obsessing about him being HIV positive and like almost as if he wanted to turn around and clean me up of that somehow, that he felt a sudden remorse or something, so I started obsessing about that. It was very strange, I felt like kind of almost disembodied and again it was kind of the sexual trance that I will sometimes go into. Uh, I just felt like I was just kind of being swept along on the events and that I was not in control of myself.
>
> *Interviewer:* How did the sex feel without a condom for you?
>
> *Jorge:* It had a kind of excitement to it but I wasn't attracted to this person so it was weird. Again I felt disembodied, like I was just swept along on events.

In the research interview, Jorge disclosed that during anonymous sexual encounters he is not totally himself, he feels "instinctual and predatory." Interestingly, this craving for anonymous sex became particularly strong when he visited his family and he had to pretend to be someone he is not.

> In that particular situation it was when I had gone home to visit my parents for the weekend and, there's something about going home that

makes me like crave sort of that anonymous outdoor sex. Uh, I pursue that uh, when I go home visiting my parents.

The disconnection between sexuality and affective life often occurs in the context of a deep longing for love, for romantic partnership, for family closeness that would not exclude sexuality. Men described many incidents and sexual episodes that were clearly disconnected from intimacy and interpersonal connection. However, those same men talked about a deep longing for intimacy, for an actual connection between their sexual and affective feelings. Like many other Latino gay men I interviewed, Jorge felt very dissatisfied with his life of sexual anonymous encounters.

> *Interviewer:* How is your sexual and personal fulfillment?
>
> *Jorge:* Um, that is like an area that I definitely don't feel satisfied with at this point. Um, I have trouble finding people who are interested in being involved on a more long-term basis. Sex I can get pretty easily but in the absence of sort of any more connection to the person it often definitely leaves a lot to be desired for me.... I can probably have as much [sex] as I want if I'm just willing to go out and look for it. But it is the lack of intimacy and connection that always concerns me and always leaves me feeling a bit empty afterwards after sex.

In addition, many Latino gay men suggested that this disconnection between sexuality and affective life was at the root of their problems with safer sex. After Manuel (fictitious name), a 31-year-old Latino gay man from Los Angeles, described one protected and another unprotected sexual encounter, the interviewer asked him to compare the two episodes. Manuel described the unprotected event in the following way:

> ... there was that sexual feeling of—that overwhelming sexual feeling. You know, it's a very kind of, you know, tactile, very sensory feeling ... it was just like this sexual frenzy, where it might have, could not have even been him, it could have been just anyone.

In those disconnected episodes, where sexuality is psychologically and effectively split off from the rest of the person's affect, cognition, and volition, partners tend to be objectified as instruments of sexual pleasure. The objectification of the partner further contributes to the lack of protection against HIV. Jorge, struggling to understand his unsafe sex encounter with someone he was not really attracted to, gave the interviewer an insightful account that relates the sexual-affect split with his loneliness, his objectification of sexual partners, and its relationship to unsafe sex.

Interviewer: What would you say were the things that led you to not use a condom that night?

Jorge: Um, more than anything else was that sense that I get when I'm in the midst of being sexually predatory of like just being very single-minded and wanting to find that person and to seduce them and to have sex with them. Um, and I think it's sort of a single-minded strange thing I feel that was happening in the left part of the brain, somehow it's not accessible to use it at that point. That was part of it. I don't know how much my down mental state had to do with it but I do know my mental state has a lot do with when I pursue sex because pursuing sex is often what I do to fill up loneliness and I know in general pursuing sex like that is about loneliness. I don't know how much not using a condom was about that. . . .

I: Was there anything about him or the specific circumstances, that setting?

J: He was very dehumanized to me. I was definitely only seeing him as someone who might be able to get me off and he was not a full human being to me. That was different from the earlier incident that I was telling you about. Part of it has to do with it being night time and not being able to see their face but also part of it is I think that it's easier to dehumanize someone for me when I don't feel like I'm really attracted to them. When I feel like I could walk away from that encounter and it wouldn't be a big loss for me or it wouldn't be difficult, I think it was a lot easier for me to dehumanize someone. When someone is attractive in whatever way you have curiosity about them, you kind of wonder with them but if you know that you're just with them to have sex and you're not even attracted to them I think they become less than human.

I: Like there won't be a romantic fantasy or desire?

J: Yeah. There won't be a romantic fantasy or desire and I don't feel obliged to take them in any way around being safe, I feel a lot less obliged to be wanting to take care of them like when I do when I'm with someone I know or like or am attracted to.

Another consequence of familism is that the building of gay community among Latino men can become a difficult endeavor. As shown by Sabogal et al. (1987), familism includes three types of value orientations: "a) perceived obligations to provide material and emotional support to the members of the extended family; b) reliance on relatives for help and support; and c) the perception of relatives as behavioral and attitudinal referents" (cited in Marin and Marin, 1991, p. 14). In other words, among Latinos, the family is seen as the main source of social support and is considered the social referent group. Thus, the notion that a group or community other than the family group could become the main source of support or referent group is somewhat alien to the Latino culture.

For many homosexual men in the Western industrialized world, support for their gay self- and social identification has been found within the context of a strongly constituted gay community, in some cases coupled with the visible presence of gay neighborhoods, gay establishments, and gay organizations. Help with coming-out issues, as well as support for working through personal shame due to internalized homophobia, is typically received in the context of membership in the gay community. Such membership, however, requires a shift of referent group from the family to the peer group, which is a re-working of social support systems and personal loyalties away from the family of origin.

I believe that the strong values of familism could present major obstacles to the sense of participation in gay community and the benefits that Latino gay men could derive from it. The shift away from support from family toward support from gay peer groups would require a deep revision of the familism value these men so deeply share. Latino gay men are often puzzled by the fact that Latino organizations and community building efforts are difficult and plagued with a great deal of interpersonal conflict and tension. It is plausible (though admittedly speculative at this time) that familism and the construction of the role of family as the ultimate referent group is one of the major obstacles to gay community building among Latino gay men. In the ideal world, we could have both family of origin and gay peer community. For the majority of Latino gay men, however, this integration of personal and family life is indeed just an ideal and, for that matter, a nearly impossible dream.

The Geographic Pseudo-Cure

A substantial number of immigrant men I talked to came to the U.S. in order to come out and live more relaxed lives as openly identified homosexuals. Many of these men were not able to deal with society's and their families' homophobia in their native countries, and chose the difficulties of exile and migration as a better—or less painful—alternative.

> *Interviewer:* How out are you in general about being gay with people you know?
>
> *Respondent:* I can say that I'm totally out, pretty out, yes.
>
> *I:* Does that include people in Mexico or only in San Francisco?
>
> *R:* It means mostly in San Francisco. In Mexico, it's funny because I consider myself out; however, it's out in parenthesis because to some people, I just don't have the need to come out to ... so I'm pretty much myself even though I sometimes might not just be talking, you know as an openly gay male.

For many other men who chose migration as a way to deal with family rejection, moving to the U.S. has not solved the problem of internalized homophobia. Once in the U.S., they may remain in the closet with co-workers and friends, see the gay community as "them," and still live their sexual lives in the context of silent, anonymous encounters. This is why I have called this particular solution to family problems the "geographic pseudo-cure." While geographic distance from the family does offer some relief and some social space for a gay life, psychological difficulties do persist in their inability for self- and public identification as homosexuals, and their inability to integrate their sexuality to their affective, emotional, and interpersonal life. There is no doubt that the strong psychological bond with the family, and its expression of loyalty through silence, transcends geographic distance.

The problems involved in the geographic pseudo-cure are evident in the interview with Carlos (fictitious name), a 28-year-old Latino gay man from San Diego. He and his Italian American lover decided to move to San Francisco a few years ago in order "to bring our [gay] life here and to be open with ourselves." Even though Carlos is open about his homosexuality with some selected members of his family, he felt an enormous amount of pressure from both his immediate and extended family in San Diego.

> My father, my grandfather, my two older sisters, my cousins, and so forth, I've never been open with them but I think maybe they probably suspect.... I feel very uncomfortable with some of my extended family.... My uncles come from a Hispanic family where it's a lot of machismo and that by this time, by 28, I should of had kids and been married, once or twice already (laughs). I go visit my distant relatives, my uncles and cousins, you know, it's really uncomfortable for them always to ask "Oh! When are you getting married? Do you have a girlfriend?" And so forth . . .

Finding a more accepting social space in San Francisco, Carlos and his lover have been able to live together and build a group of friends that can respect them and treat them as who they are, a gay couple. At different times during the interview, however, it was clear that Carlos is still experiencing in San Francisco many of the difficulties originally created by the silence kept in loyalty to his family. For example, Carlos sees his life with a gay partner primarily as a "sexual" choice rather than as a family of his own choosing, and hence a personal "private" matter, rather than a social identity:

> for me, I'm still pretty private. If someone will ask me outright if I'm gay, I will answer them correctly. . . . However, I think your sexual life is your private life.

Disclosure of his homosexuality and talk about his gay partner is difficult for Carlos, even among friends who obviously know he is gay. This was especially true with gay friends who now live in San Francisco but had some connections to his San Diego family.

> ...these friends are from our family and friends in San Diego, so when we all kind of got together in San Francisco they knew who I was. I was

gay and that I lived with my partner but it took a little while for us all to openly discuss our relationships.

Now in San Francisco, living happily with his lover, Carlos still has problems staying away from sexual anonymous encounters and public sex environments. In his view, those encounters were his only possible sexual outlets while living in the context of his family in San Diego.

> There have been a few times when my partner is out of town and I've gone to an adult bookstore and just kind of not flirted but just kind of to see what was there because that used to be, not my life per se, but that was the extent of my sexual experience which now, when I look back on, is nothing I would ever want to do again because I'm so happy with who I am with now. A few times I've been there just to see what happens and I find out it's not what I want but there's always that, not drive but kind of inkling, what if? What if?
>
> *Interviewer:* So when you have been to the bookstores in the past year have you allowed yourself to become sexually involved with any of these men there?
>
> *Carlos:* Mm, once, well a few times maybe. It was just basically touch and that's about it, but once I did go back to a hotel with one person.

As he had predicted, the interview transcript reveals that Carlos has difficulties talking about his "private" sexual life. Unfortunately, this difficulty in communication about sexual matters also happens with his lover, his primary sexual partner, creating a difficult and risky situation from the point of view of HIV transmission. Carlos and his lover have negotiated safety from HIV by agreeing not to use condoms within their monogamous relationship. Carlos occasionally slips from his monogamy agreement and wonders whether his partner does also. In addition, Carlos has been tested for HIV with negative results, but his partner has never been tested. Even though his own situation worries Carlos immensely, and his waiting for the HIV test results every six months is typically an agonizing experience, communication between him and his partner about these matters is virtually nil.

> [AIDS] could happen to anybody but when it comes to that point, you know, it's like there's no way I'll take the risk. This is a difficult subject

because it's something I'm going through right now where I'm not just
as open with my partner about some of these topics I'm discussing now
so it's a little difficult. I've been dealing with this whole issue for about a
year already where it's really aggravating to me. . . .

Interviewer: So, you are still uncertain of your partner's HIV status. Is
 that right?

Carlos: That's correct. As far as I know he hasn't been tested and I have
 not really—it was brought up about two years ago, actually three
 years, and it was kind of avoided.

Carlos' silence about sexual matters, originally developed as a coping
mechanism to deal with family rejection of homosexuality, is deeply
internalized. The sexual silence has come with him to San Francisco
and, while no longer adaptive, such silence has become perhaps his
major vulnerability to HIV infection.

The Many Faces of Sexual Silence

I was struck and somewhat puzzled, especially during the focus-group
interviews, by the difficulties men experienced when talking openly
about sex. More often than not, men spoke about their sexual experiences without explicit reference to specific sexual activities, that is,
they either became silent or strongly hesitated when they needed to
use sex words. An example of this difficulty can be seen in the moving
story of one focus-group participant who told the group about his sexual initiation around the age of seven with an older man, a friend of
the family. After explaining the different contextual elements of the
story, the sexual act was described with the following phrase: *"y cuando
pasó lo que tenia que pasar"* ("and when what needed to happen happened"). Similarly, especially among men of Mexican origin, the word
"relaciones" ("relations") was often used to describe sex: *"tuvimos relaciones"* ("we had relations"), meaning "we had sex." During the interviews, men often paused, apologized, or giggled with embarrassment at
explicit words that describe sexual practices.

In line with the behavior observed during the interviews, men often
expressed difficulties in talking about sex with casual partners. Men
discussed how frequently, even though it was very much on their
minds, the topics of condoms and limitations on sexual practices were

difficult to discuss or not discussed openly with their potential sexual partners. When I inquired about the use of condoms in casual sex, a man described a pick-up at a Latino gay bar that ended in an unprotected sexual encounter saying *"y de eso, ni se habló"* ("and of that, we didn't even talk")—"that" in reference to condom use.

It seems that, outside the domain of jokes or boasting about conquests, serious discussions about sexuality are extremely difficult and rare among Latino gay men. These observations are consistent with recent survey findings regarding high rates of "sexual discomfort" among Latinos, and findings regarding the silence about sexuality found within Latino families (Baumeister, Flores, and Marín, 1995; CDC, 1991; Padilla, 1987). Sexual silence, especially about homosexuality, is not surprising in light of the observations about homophobia within Latino families. As discussed in the previous section, acceptance of homosexuality within Latino families can be achieved only if it remains underground, not talked about, "under the carpet"; silence about sexuality is no doubt a most efficient way to keep shameful behavior under the carpet of public discourse and removed as much as possible from the world of conscious reality.

Sexual silence can be understood also in light of a well-recognized Latino value known as *Simpatía*, which expresses the importance of smooth, conflict-free, and non-confrontative interpersonal relations. In the words of Marín and Marín (1991):

> *Simpatía* emphasizes the need for behaviors that promote smooth and pleasant social relationships. As a script, *simpatía* moves the individual to show a certain level of conformity and empathy for the feelings of other people. In addition, a person with *simpatía* (*simpático*) behaves with dignity and respect towards others and strives to achieve harmony in interpersonal relations. Researchers have operationally defined *simpatía* as a general tendency toward avoiding interpersonal conflict, emphasizing positive behaviors in agreeable situations, and de-emphasizing negative behaviors in conflictive circumstances. (p. 12)

Because conversations about sexuality can bring to the surface potentially embarrassing, sensitive or private matters of individuals, the Latino *simpatía* script promotes silence rather than open and frank discussion about sexuality. I believe *simpatía* is directly relevant to understanding the lack of discussion about safe sex practices, especially between casual sex partners. Many men in the interviews mentioned that asking their partners to use condoms felt very uncomfortable because they were afraid that their partners would get offended. Apparently, these men were concerned that the request for condom use would be interpreted by their partners as an accusation of being promiscuous, infected, or sick. In many cases, acting *simpático* toward a desirable potential sex partner, especially an unfamiliar person, and protecting their partners from uncomfortable feelings seemed to take precedence over protection from HIV infection.

I have often wondered why the sexual silence exists—that is, why is it that sexuality is such a difficult topic for open discussion among Latinos, especially within the context of the family. I would like to state my current thinking as hypotheses that need to be validated with further systematic observations.

There are at least three facts of our communities that are not particularly a source of cultural pride among Latinos: a high frequency of homosexual and bisexual behavior among men who identify as heterosexuals, a high incidence of sexual abuse or sexual initiation of relatively young children by older relatives or family friends, and a high incidence of marital infidelity with the justification that men need to find sexual release with multiple partners and that it would be "unmanly" to resist any female advances. It is possible that these three facts are considered "ugly" or "dirty laundry" by the culture, and need to be kept outside the realm of public discourse and awareness, especially in light of the *simpatía* script. It would be almost impossible for the culture to initiate an open dialogue about sexuality without confronting these three major facts that for so long have been kept under the carpet in the name of *simpatía* among respectful families and individuals.

It is precisely the denial of these three problems—sexual abuse, bisexuality, and marital infidelity—with which the AIDS epidemic has confronted our culture. I believe that little progress in AIDS prevention within the Latino community will be made until we are willing to break the sexual silence and discuss openly, with dignity and compassion, the reality of our sexual lives and the factors that may prevent our further spreading the AIDS virus. In the meantime, Latino gay men are especially at risk to the extent that they participate in the culture and are willing to conspire with the silence. Needless to say, the by now familiar phrase "Silence = Death" is especially relevant to the Latino community.

Impact on Perceptions of Sexual Control

Perhaps the deepest effect of sexual silence is the actual inability to access sexuality or sexual feelings in a cognitive, analytical manner. Silence splits off sexuality from cognition to the extent that thinking processes, as well as attempts at regulatory control, are seen as incompatible with sexual arousal. When describing the difficulties he had with condoms, one of the men interviewed described how the mere act of thinking he had to use a condom interrupted the flow of events during a sexual encounter.

> Here we are, in the foreplay, getting hotter and hotter in preparation for penetration and then all of a sudden I say, oh condoms! Where are they? Where did you put them? And by the time I think where they are and look for them, I lose interest, I lose my erection, and tell my partner, can we do this tomorrow?

Thus, the perceptions of low sexual control I encountered in many men I interviewed also involved a belief in the incompatibility between thinking processes and sexual arousal. This incompatibility was reflected in one man's distinction between "participants" and "spectators" in a sexual encounter.

> When you think about the need to use condoms, you become a spectator, and you can't participate. You can't be both, you are either a participant or a spectator.

The distinction between spectator and participant roles for people who are actual participants in a sexual act is a troublesome one, especially when it equates regulatory awareness or control with the spectator role. The underlying mental representation is that any attempt at controlling or regulating the sexual encounter will lead to a psychological distancing from the situation and a consequent loss of physical and psychological sexual arousal. Needless to say, when taken to its ultimate consequences, this perception or belief constitutes a major psychological barrier to the practice of safer sex among "passionate" Latino gay men.

In Conclusion

It may seem puzzling or paradoxical that I have discussed the family as a source of risk when, for Latinos as a whole, the family constitutes a protective factor against the stresses of poverty and minority status. However, when one considers the implications of familism for Latino homosexuals—namely, internalized homophobia, a sense of personal shame, the separation of sexuality and affective life, and the lack of a gay peer referent group—then it becomes clear how such cultural values might be strongly related to difficulties in the practice of safe sex. Research has shown that difficulties in coming out and a lack of social support are predictors of high risk practices (Catania, Coates, and Stall, 1991; Catania et al., 1991; Coates et al., 1988). The time has come to examine how some of these predictors may be closely tied to the shared beliefs and values about the importance of family life, when defined in heterosexual terms.

It is important to end this chapter, however, noting that not all Latino families can be considered homophobic and that great variability exists in the Latino community regarding the degree of family acceptance of their children's homosexuality. Similarly, there is great variability in how many and how much Latino gay men have been able to integrate their sexual and affective lives by dealing with internalized homophobia, participating in gay culture, and creating gay families. The gay liberation movement has indeed developed, though with many difficulties, in Latin America (see, e.g., Carrier, 1989; Lumsden, 1991) and in the U.S. Latino community. With it, Latino gay organizations have begun to emerge in major urban cities, promoting and supporting their members' coming-out process and its consequences for family life. Nonetheless, from the interviews I have conducted so far, it is my impression that Latino gay men still feel pretty isolated, don't feel part of a community, and have difficulties participating in gay events and other community-building activities. More important, the relationship to family is still highly problematic for most of us, and the consequences of family conflict mentioned above are still highly prevalent.

Invariably, men who spoke with pride about their homosexuality and seemed well connected to the gay community were men who had spoken openly to their families and either experienced acceptance or consciously walked away from the family with a sense of personal dignity. Above all, it was clear to me that, for many Latino gay men, the homophobic conflict with *la familia* was very much at the root of high-risk sexual practices.

6.

Poverty and Racism

The Fueling of Fatalism

> I get tested somewhere around yearly and when I get a nega-
> tive result I feel relieved, I feel happy. I feel like each of them
> is like, OK. Here. You get another x–period of time. . . . And
> that's kind of a fatalism I think cuz' it feels like OK. I'm OK.
> for now.
>
> —30-year-old Latino gay man

In a recent study of Latino gay and bisexual men in San Francisco, we asked respondents to estimate their likelihood of becoming infected in the future. The question, addressed only to HIV-negative men in the sample, was stated as follows: "What do you think are your chances of becoming HIV positive in the future?" The four possible responses ranged from *none* and *low* to *medium* and *high*. Even though only a few men responded "high," much to our surprise, only about 10 percent of HIV negative men in the sample were able to give an unequivocal *none* response. This survey question had been used before to assess perceived vulnerability to HIV among gay and bisexual men. My sense is that, in our study, we actually tapped men's fatalism regarding the inevitability of HIV infection. Latino men's responses suggested not only that they indeed feel very vulnerable to HIV but also that such an outcome might be well beyond their own sense of personal control.

Similar fatalistic themes of inevitability emerged in the focus groups and individual interviews; the sense that HIV infection is unavoidable, that it would happen to them sooner or later, was expressed by different men in many different ways. Some men talked about AIDS as *el premio gordo* (the grand price), alluding to their belief that luck in life's lottery, rather than risky behavior, is the ultimate cause of infection. Some men talked about their belief that changes in behavior that transmit HIV could only happen through the effort of several generations, assuming that the task of changing sexual behavior is beyond the capacity of individuals and too big for any one individual to undertake. These men saw themselves as impotent in the face of HIV, placing their hope for the community in the effort of "younger ones," not aware that many younger men felt exactly their same sense of impotence. Others talked about a diffuse sense of fate where HIV is only one of the multiple adversities they face in life, over which they have little control: "If it's going to happen, it will" or *"Si te va a tocar, no hay nada que puedas hacer"* (If it's going to happen to you, there's nothing you can do).

In other fields of public health, researchers have documented the presence of fatalism among Latinos and its negative effects on mobilizing individuals to take preventive measures vis-à-vis preventable outcomes. For example, in a study of attitudes and beliefs about cancer, Pérez-Stable et al. (1995) found that about half of their Latino sample believed that receiving a cancer diagnosis is equivalent to "getting a death sentence." Also, they found that a higher proportion of Latinos (26%) than non-Latino Whites (18%) believed that there is little one can do to prevent the disease.

There is no doubt that fatalism—the belief that fate dictates life (including health) outcomes, and that fate is basically unbeatable (Ferriss, 1993)—is highly prevalent among Latinos, and to a higher degree than in the non-Latino White population. As reporter Susan Ferriss bluntly stated, fatalism is itself a health threat for Latinos.

While the roots of Latino fatalism have been attributed to several long standing sources of oppression, ranging from the influence of the Catholic Church to generations of economic and political repression in Latin America, researchers and scholars typically refer to it as a trait or characteristic of the Hispanic/Latino culture. Identifying fatalism as a cultural theme, trait, or characteristic, however, does little to guide our HIV-prevention strategies with Latino gay men. In order to serve our purpose and further our understanding of the situation of Latino gay men in the AIDS epidemic in this country, I want to explore several themes that emerged from qualitative interviews powerfully linking poverty, racism, and the risk for HIV. These themes illuminate the fact that HIV fatalism among Latino gay men is not merely an exaggerated or culturally distorted perception of risk, but rather a perception of personal and collective vulnerability fueled by experiences of poverty and racism.

It is important to recognize that poverty and racism are not only experienced externally or "out there" but also that they leave undeniable internalized scars in those who are oppressed. Fatalism regarding health outcomes is a clear indicator of such internalization. I want, therefore, to examine fatalism regarding HIV infection not just as a cultural characteristic of Latino gay men but also as a meaningful cognitive construction that emerges from specific experiences of social disempowerment, also experienced and manifested in the sexual domain.

It is important to examine closely the impact of poverty and racism specifically on the *sexual* lives of Latino gay men. While many public health studies have investigated the impact of race and socioeconomic status on morbidity and mortality across a wide range of diseases, including AIDS, it is not clear how the experiences of poverty and racism affect individuals' abilities to regulate their own sexuality. This lack of understanding is distressing given the fact that HIV is not randomly distributed among the population and its continued spread in the U.S. occurs mostly within social and geographical boundaries defined by poverty and minority status.

Above all, I want to portray fatalism not as a cultural or personal deficit, nor as a distorted Latino cognition, but rather as a meaningful perception from the perspective of those whose lives unfold in the midst of poverty and racism. In other words, I want to show that there is a certain element of truth in the fatalistic perceptions of Latino gay men. These men are involved in contexts larger and more powerful than themselves, and over which they have little control. It is precisely those disempowering contexts, created mostly by poverty and racism, that undermine the self-regulation and self-determination of sexual behavior. It is in those contexts that both fatalism and HIV mutually reinforce their existence.

Poor, Brown, and Gay

First, I must bring to the forefront the fact that Latinos in the U.S., gay men included, are disproportionately stricken by poverty, racism, and sociopolitical alienation. In fact, from 1979 to 1992 Latino poverty rates increased by six percentage points, as compared to one point for African Americans and 1.6 points for non-Latino Whites (Enchautegui, 1995). In addition, the recent and quite strong anti-immigrant sentiment in the country, represented by the popularity of Proposition 187 in California, witnesses the increasing racial intolerance toward individuals and groups of Latino descent. Proposition 187 was crafted mostly to withhold and deny health, education, and social services to Mexican undocumented immigrants and their families, even though undocumented workers from Mexico contribute substantially to California's economy and pay their fair share of state and federal taxes.

The fact is that the overwhelming majority of Latino immigrants to the U.S.—including gay men—are gradually assimilated *not* into a mainstream culture of wealth and possibility (the so-called American Dream) but rather into a caste-like, disadvantaged minority status that not only is self-perpetuating but also conspires against the whole purpose of immigration for a healthier, financially stable, and socially safe life. Such breakdown of immigration goals and dreams is powerfully portrayed in the film *El Norte* (The North), where two Guatemalan political refugees encounter the most devastating consequences of poverty not in rural Guatemala but in the midst of urban Los Angeles as exploited undocumented workers.

Latino gay men develop their sense of self in a social context characterized by triple oppression: poverty, racism, and homophobia. Even though as social scientists we can analyze separately the effects of these three sources of oppression, Latino gay men have subjectively experienced *one* history of prejudice, discrimination, and social alienation. Being poor, brown, and gay are deeply intertwined in an overwhelming sense of being different, for which they have been terribly rejected and abused. For many men I interviewed, it was clear that being brown and being poor went together. Many others confessed that often it was not clear whether the laughter, teasing, or social alienation from other classmates was because they were gay (e.g., they liked to play with girls more than boys), or because they looked different, or because they lived on the wrong side of the tracks.

> I think I've always felt different, yeah!, even from the other kids that were different. I think I was just a little more different. At that age when

you are young, a child, I don't think you have a way to describe that feeling of difference but you know that [it] exists. Not only was I not like the other Anglo kids, I was Mexican, I was brown, which meant that I was poor and lived in those areas. And that was true, all the other kids around me I saw having a fairly good standard of living in their homes. In my home it was pretty much hand-to-mouth and later on I began to realize that a lot of what we considered luxuries was commonplace with these other folks, and they didn't live, but maybe two blocks down the street from me. It made me probably just a little sad I guess. I don't think anger came into it yet, because I didn't have an analysis of the economic situation. In that sense I was different, different in the sense that I preferred to play with the girls rather than playing with the boys, even more so. People couldn't pinpoint me in any particular category.

Being gay and being brown have been also negatively paired in encounters with the law around sexual activity in public places. Men in the study related instances where they were unjustly insulted, harassed, and even arrested by policemen who accused them unjustly of sexual misconduct. Men who had been arrested or harassed by the police in connection to homosexual activity were convinced that their being Latino was the decisive variable in the harassment or arrest.

I had just turned 18, and I was arrested with somebody that was, he was late 17, and we had fucked in the hills in Hillsborough, in the car, and the police came by. They didn't catch us doing anything, but they charged me with contributing delinquency of a minor, and indecent exposure. . . . I was prosecuted and yeah, it actually hit me because I wasn't caught doing anything. The truth is, yes, I did have sex. . . . It wasn't that we were in public doing this, but it's the prejudice I'm sure. Then there was the time I was with a friend and we stopped, we took turns going to the bathroom, so I'm there taking a leak and this little guy, happens to be Latin, comes in, stands next to me and he is chatty, we didn't have any sexual interests, anyway, there was nothing going on, I'm not here to do anything, there is nothing I can do there, I'm not going to sit there and play with myself, I don't, anyway the police come in and he, wang, wang wang, "put your hands up against the wall," arrested me for loitering and intention of committing a lewd and lascivious act. . . . I guess I can actually say that I've experienced both prejudices, for being gay and Latin. . . . I've had the police call me names just for being Latin.

The convergence of poverty, racism, and homophobia is particularly obvious in the case of *Vestidas*, literally, "the ones who dress up" (note feminine ending -as), used as an umbrella term for Latino transvestive-transgender individuals in San Francisco. In my qualitative study, I had one focus group for *Vestidas* from the San Francisco Latino Mission district; all the participants of this particular focus group turned out to be unemployed, surviving minimally through disability checks for AIDS diagnoses or through prostitution work. *Vestidas* complained about their inability to find a "proper" job and having to "work the streets" in order to eat, especially after they had adopted a feminine identity and begun to dress up as women on a daily basis. Even though many *Vestidas* I interviewed were quite articulate, competent, and some had professional degrees from their native countries, they could not find employment within Latino establishments. In addition, because all of them were immigrants and had difficulties with the English language, finding jobs in the mainstream business world, or even within the mainstream gay community, was out of the question.

A large proportion of immigrant *Vestidas* become prostitutes in order to survive. However, it is important to note also that prostitution is a culturally sanctioned profession for men who dress up as women. *Vestidas* who become prostitutes have the added incentive that heterosexually identified men who want to have sex with men often do so with *Vestidas* who are prostitutes. Often these "straight" men verbally abuse them and beat them up as a way to alleviate their homosexual anxiety after having sex with them. *Vestida* prostitutes are often the target of police harrassment that involves strong racist elements. Some of them complained about the fact that police harassment makes carrying condoms a very difficult endeavor. To the police, the presence of condoms in the *Vestidas'* purses would be treated as a confession or evidence of prostitution.

Thus, it is not possible to understand the HIV risk of Latino homosexual men in this country without an awareness that these men are also an "ethnic minority" and experience their sexuality in a context characterized by poverty, racial prejudice, and social inequality. In fact, quite often, Latino gay men experience being gay, poor, and an ethnic minority as a single experience of being different, abused, and disadvantaged. When you are discriminated against for being brown, poor, and gay, it is not possible to separate your developing sexual identity from the disempowering experiences of poverty and racism.

Powerful Others

A consistent theme across the focus groups and individual interviews was the notion that somewhere out there is a group of powerful others that are responsible for multiple negative outcomes in the lives of Latino gay and bisexual men, including the spread of HIV. Many men used a vaguely defined pronoun "they" or talk about "them" with the strong conviction that there are socially, financially, and politically powerful authority figures that determine their well-being, including their individual HIV risk.

The vaguely defined "them" was used often in reference to individuals, groups, and institutions that do in fact have enormous power and control over the lives of many men I interviewed. "Them" are employers who pay below the minimum wage, social service workers who ask humiliating questions, health care providers who seem to blame rather than understand, White gay men whose overeager interest in Spanish accents make them feel both attractive and uncomfortable, and, of course, immigration officials. In specific reference to the spread of HIV, "them" would be Catholic priests who refuse to talk about condoms in their Sunday sermons or epidemiologists from the San Francisco Department of Health who write up confusing safer sex guidelines; in many other cases, however, "they" would neither be named nor defined. "They," nonetheless, were seen as having enormous power in determining individuals' HIV risk. "They" were blamed or given credit, but never really trusted.

The main point is that, in the minds of many men I interviewed, especially the immigrant and the poor, HIV is only one of the multiple adversities they face and over which they have little control. In fact, most of the adverse realities these men face in their daily lives do stem from financial, social, and political dependencies on powerful others. Why should HIV be otherwise? From lack of privacy in congested housing quarters to hours of painful time in the overcrowded waiting rooms of public hospitals, the experiences of actual dependence on powerful others have fostered a sense of helplessness and hopelessness in many Latino gay men I interviewed.

Helplessness vis-à-vis adversity is coped with mostly by the development of a refined and acute sense of fate. The notion of fate, and the resulting fatalistic perception of life, is constructed as an explanation that gives meaning and offers relief from situations that otherwise would breed frustration and rage. Somehow it is easier and more soothing to believe that hours of waiting in pain at the public hospital are "meant to be," rather than deal with the sense of anger, powerlessness, and humiliation provoked by the insensitivity and disrespect of overworked health care workers who make you feel they are doing you a big favor for treating your illness or pain.

Psychologists have proposed the construct "locus of control" as a personality dimension or orientation based on individuals' belief about the controllability of events in their lives (see, e.g., Rotter, 1971). An "external" (in contrast to an "internal") locus of control describes individuals who believe they do not have control over the events that regulate their lives. An external locus of control is thus a form of fatalism, ingrained somehow in the cognitive schemata and personality structure of individuals who have the trait. Persons with an external locus of control have difficulties in self-regulation.

I believe that many of the Latino gay men I interviewed, if tested, would score very high on measures of external locus of control. However, more than a reflection of a quasi-pathological construction, the measure would reflect the realistic perceptions and cognitive constructions of those who are the victims of poverty and racism. The real tragedy lies in the fact that once such a sense of externality is created, it becomes a filter through which all outcomes, positive or negative, controllable or uncontrollable, are perceived. In other words, the problem is not that fatalism is a hazardous cultural trait of Latinos but that its truthfulness and meaning are over-generalized to situations that can be potentially controlled, such as in the case of HIV transmission.

In the context of a fatalistic orientation to life—an orientation that is repeatedly reinforced by experiences of dependence on powerful others—it is a bit naive to train people in self-efficacy for safer sexual behavior, as if the notion of personal power or control over life events is a skill to be learned within a weekend safer sex workshop. It is not possible simply to show HIV as a different kind of adversity that "Yes, you can" control it (or some other version of "Just say no" or the even more ridiculous "Just don't do it") without understanding that multiple experiences of poverty and racism in daily life reinforce the opposite feeling. How can we expect individuals who have little control over most of their lives' events to act with a great deal of agency and self-efficacy in the practice of safer sex? To believe that we can treat sexuality as a different and disconnected domain from individuals' lives is perhaps the biggest mistake of those who advocate HIV prevention from a behavioristic or cognitive-behavioral perspective, focusing in a narrow-minded fashion on the eroticization of condoms, sexual negotiation skills, or self-efficacy for safer sex. Epidemiological findings are hitting us in the head with the following truth: HIV transmission is not only a disease but also a symptom, a marker of poverty and discrimination. We have been too slow to incorporate this lesson in our HIV prevention efforts.

Powerless Selves

My research suggests that experiences of poverty and dependence become internalized as a deeply felt sense of individual powerlessness and fatalism regarding life outcomes, including health status. This sense of powerlessness becomes over-generalized to situations where some control could be potentially exercised. Thus, as in the case of internalized machismo, our own internalized oppression conspires with the devastating effects of poverty and racism in our lives.

Nowhere is internalized oppression more evident than in the characterization of "Latinos" and "Latino gay men" given by those I interviewed. In contrast to powerful others, who are perceived as having the knowledge and power to stop the epidemic, men saw themselves and their referent groups as powerless individuals, as some sort of *manadas* (herds) that act in a sheeplike, other-directed fashion.

In the words of Victor, one of the Latino gay activists I interviewed:

> ... *estamos acostumbrados a vivir como manadas. La gente le echa la culpa a los mas grandes, los políticos, la religión, otros. Pero no se dice, "hasta aquí llegó esto; yo tomo la decisión ..."* (We are accustomed to live like herds. People blame the big ones [powerful others], politicians, religion, others. But we never say, "this needs to stop here; I make the decision...")

The internalized scars of poverty and racism, manifested in negative self-perceptions of powerlessness and incompetence, were nowhere more visible than in research participants' views of the Latino community and of Latino gay men vis-à-vis the HIV epidemic. When I asked participants to speak about the barriers to HIV prevention, many of them mentioned that it was very difficult for Latino gay men to organize themselves or attend organized groups. On the one hand, many men recognized that other life problems—unemployment, inadequate housing, substance abuse, violence—were more pressing and did not allow much free time for activities other than finding daily sustenance and surviving in an often hostile society. On the other hand, men also spoke of Latinos as truly disempowered, that is, unable to see beyond their own immediate needs and mobilize together with their communities to solve the problems that face them, including HIV. A major complaint was that Latinos, they believe, expect others to solve their problems.

> *Los Latinos tratamos de venir a este país para progresar y sobrevvir, y a veces no tenemos el tiempo para hacer grupos, ya que hay que trabajar muy duro para comer. Y este es uno de los factores por la que no hay tanta organización Latina. Otra es que estamos esperando que se nos resuelva el problema o estamos esperando algún beneficio personal, y si vemos que no, nos retiramos.* (We Latinos come to this country to progress and survive, and many times we do not have the time to do groups because we have to work so hard in order to eat. And this is one of the reasons why there are so few Latino organizations. The other thing is that we are waiting for someone else to solve our problems, or we are expecting some personal benefit, and if we see there isn't, we remove ourselves.)
>
> *¿Cuál es la diferencia entre la comunidad Latina y la comunidad blanca? . . . Los americanos son más activistas, los Latinos esperan que todo se lo resuelva otros.* (What is the difference between the Latino and the White community? . . . Americans are more activist, Latinos are waiting for someone else to solve all their problems.)

Latinos were seen as unable to organize themselves for HIV prevention work, lacking not only time but also social conscience. Latinos were portrayed as envious because of issues of class and education, involved in their own problems out of self-interest, and unable to commit their time to community-relevant projects.

The following comments were made about the problem of recruiting enough Latino volunteers for San Francisco's Shanti Project:

> si el Latino se hace voluntario es por sacar algo o por curiosidad. De los 15 que tomaron el curso quedan sólo tres. (If a Latino becomes a volunteer, it's only to get something out of it, or because he is curious. Of the 15 that took the [volunteer] training, only three remain.)

Men talked about how Latinos' inhibition, embarrassment, and fear interfered even with the ability to do role plays in safer sex workshops. "Somos miedosos para pararnos en un escenario, nos da pena." (We are scared to step on a stage, we feel embarrassed). Many felt that we deal with our inhibition and fear by using alcohol and drugs rather than face the realities of our lives in a problem-solving manner.

It was interesting, but also very painful, to witness that even when I directly asked participants about the limitations of HIV prevention efforts targeting Latino gay men, they would often blame themselves rather than the programs. They would blame Latino men's inability to organize, their being caught up in self-interest, as well as their inhibition and fear. Their self-blame regarding the inability to deal with the challenges brought about by the AIDS epidemic, instead of confronting the ineffective prevention programs, echoed their self-blame in hurting their families for being gay.

The men I interviewed seemed to be caught in a tragic bind—a life regulated by the oppression of powerful others on the one hand, and the inability of perceived powerless, defective selves to take charge of their own lives on the other. In fact, Latino gay men spoke about themselves in ways that many of us would not tolerate others to talk about our community. As the interviews progressed, the deprecatory caricature-like perceptions about being Latino sounded to me more and more like instances of internalized racism. The self-perceptions of powerlessness and incompetence witnessed for me in a most dramatic fashion the internalized scars of *both* poverty and racism in our communities. For many Latino gay men, especially the more acculturated ones, such internalized self-deprecation is reinforced by frequent experiences of racism within the gay community.

Racism in the Gay Community

Many English-speaking Latino gay men, perhaps to get away from the devastating effects of homophobia, poverty, and racism in their native communities, spend a considerable amount of time, resources, and effort attempting to fit in and develop a sense of belonging to a mainstream, mostly White and middle class, gay community. Although I found deprecatory comments about Latinos in both acculturated and non-acculturated men, only the English-speaking, more acculturated men seemed to deal with the issues by moving away from Latino environments and attempting to integrate themselves into the mainstream gay community. They often found themselves, however, rejected or alienated because of racist attitudes among gay men. At times, they seemed to live in two different worlds: the Latino community and the gay community. However, the experience of many acculturated Latino gay men I interviewed was one of social alienation, of not belonging to either the Latino *or* the gay community. Some men seemed to move from city to city, from job to job, from apartment to apartment, trying to find a sense of community they so profoundly thirsted for. The feeling was one of being in a disorienting social state of flux.

> I think that you hit the nail on the head when you said earlier that often times gay Latino men are disjointed from our communities, I think I feel the same way. I've always had, it seems, and it may just be my background. I don't belong here, I don't belong there, and I'm supposed to try to fit somewhere, but when you see that acceptance is not forthcoming . . . it's kind of being in a state of flux. I think that's really influenced a lot of my decisions about work and living situations, not always for the better though.

Racism in the gay community ranges from blatant discrimination to experiences of feeling invisible when relating to men who search for Latin lovers. Not surprisingly, I found many of the acculturated men truly angry and disappointed at their attempts to fit in.

> I hate the Castro, I can't stand it. It is a ghetto, people should wear pink stars. Financially well-off white, it is so closed!! If you are male and white yes there is a gay community. All the programs are run by the middle-class gay men . . . a lot of prejudices in the gay community.

To many Latino gay men who purposefully come to San Francisco in search of a gay haven of tolerance and acceptance, the experience of racism in the gay community can be devastating. As one of the men told me, "I found more racism in the Castro than in Minnesota." Another participant echoed similar feelings:

> I think in the Castro, it was the one place I felt a little less comfortable, but I kept going back because it was the gay place and people, we would run into friends, etc., but I felt less attractive there, a lot of times I felt like I was the only wonder who wasn't white, and you know that's true . . . at that time I remember the I.D. policy also. If they really didn't want you there, they come to the door and say "3 I.D. policy," against men-of-color and against women.

Many acculturated men immerse themselves into the mainstream gay community as a way of leaving behind the machismo and homophobia of their own communities, such as Latino definitions of homosexuality as a gender issue, discussed in Chapter 4. Much to their surprise, they encounter the same attitudes in the racist stereotypes of White gay men whose fascination with Latinos only perpetuates the cultural oppression.

> My brothers were more abusive, when I got to the age that I was supposed to do the things that machos are supposed to do, I was pegged from age 5. Growing with this kind of self-image it is kind of devastating, you know, being gay and coming to the white gay community you were expected to be either a drag queen or a macho type.

Through my research, I have witnessed many stories of sexual encounters where Latino gay men were objectified by White gay men who sought fantasies of the "exotic, dark, and passionate" flavor. On one hand, the fantasies were extremely seductive to acculturated men because they were, above all, thirsty for acceptance by, recognition from, and a sense of belonging with other gay men. On the other hand, the White gay men's fantasies reinforced their feelings of deficiency fostered by the machismo in the culture. Now, within the gay community, the oppression seemed only worse. Through those fantasy-like sexual events, Latino gay men were now experiencing oppression from the peer group they so badly expected acceptance from:

I think that the dynamics that sometimes go on between Anglo men and Latinos is one that they may come to Latinos looking for a top man to fuck them, and a lot of it has to do with power, power over . . . working relationships. Going into this situation thinking "this is my hot Latin lover," another phrase I've heard a lot.

Not surprisingly, Latino gay men are very ambivalent about the attraction White gay men have for them. On one hand, they feel flattered for the attention they receive; on the other hand, they realize that the attraction is not about them but about a fantasy they represent.

I guess I like Anglos, not to say that I wouldn't go out with Latinos. I guess a lot of Anglo men are attracted to me because I'm Latino. Sometimes I have a problem with that. Sometimes it feels kind of nice that someone is interested in me because I'm Latino, and sometimes they have a lot of expectations, like hot men in bed . . . totally very sexual, totally very passionate. . . . I know that I'm passionate not because I'm Latino, but because I've dated men and a lot of them were passionate anyway. Anglos are attracted to me because I'm Latino but I like that. I like to get attention, and I don't want to seem conceited because men are attracted to me. But I would say that Latinos aren't attracted to me. Some of them are, but Anglos pay more attention to me, and they pick me out in the crowd when they look around. And I like it, and I don't think it's bad. The thing that bothers me the most is when Anglos have that attitude that says I only go out with Latinos. That's when I feel very uncomfortable with that kind of statement, for them being a little more attracted to me because I'm Latin. That's OK, but I want them to be also attracted to me because of the way I am.

In Summary

In the two preceding chapters, I discussed how machismo, homophobia, family loyalty, and sexual silence—as forces that shape the lives and sexuality of Latino gay men—conspire to undermine perceptions of sexual control. In this chapter, I have discussed two other factors, poverty and racism, that join the conspiracy. In the context of poverty and racism, however, perceptions of sexual control become less and less accessible. More than simply a perception of low control, poverty and racism promote a sense of fatalism, an external locus of control where life, sexuality, and health are at the mercy of powerful others and ultimately fate that, by definition, is beyond our power to control.

Men's deeply internalized fatalism is constantly being reinforced by *actual* experiences of powerlessness vis-à-vis social institutions and powerful others that regulate their lives as well as their sexuality. In particular, the sexual contexts created by poverty and racism—contexts of financial dependence, racially motivated power dynamics, and an over-riding thirst for acceptance and inclusion—present enormous obstacles to exercising actual control and self-regulation over sexual behavior. If the perception of self-efficacy for safer sex behavior is the main psychological predictor of behavior change, I would venture to say that the actual cultural and social context of Latino gay men's lives constitutes a breeding ground for HIV. This tragic breeding ground is shared particularly by those in our society who are simultaneously oppressed by homophobia, poverty, and racism. Isn't this what epidemiological findings of who is HIV infected in the U.S. are telling us?

7.

Acculturation Groups

Our target population of Latino gay men constitutes a diverse group of men that vary in a number of important variables such as age, socioeconomic status, education, nationality, race, degree of gay identification, and level of integration to the mainstream, English-speaking society. It is admittedly difficult to make and discuss generalizable statements about Latino gay men as a well-defined population. Nonetheless, beyond the individual differences and heterogeneous nature of this group, there are important sources of commonality among Latino gay men, especially in areas of relevance and concern to AIDS education and prevention.

Chapters 4, 5, and 6 focused on cultural values and experiences shared by most, if not all, Latino gay men. There is, for example, the shared experience of growing up homosexual in a society that values strong adherence to rigidly defined sex roles and where males, from a very young age, are asked and encouraged to prove their masculinity through risk taking and sexual prowess. There is a set of shared influences and shared values that cut across nationalities and socioeconomic groups, such as the strong influence of the Catholic Church and the life-long intense involvement of parents, siblings, and relatives in the lives and decisions of individual members of the family. Last, but not least, the shared Spanish language and Hispanic culture offer important sources of commonality in the form of popular proverbs, sayings, songs, and shared meanings that shape to a large extent a common world view and a set of shared values (Marín and Marín, 1991). Our task is thus to consider both sources of diversity and commonality, taking into account that it does make some sense to talk about Latino gay men in the U.S. as a coherent, though diverse group of men.

A useful way to define Latino gay men in both their diversity and commonality is to consider the existence of naturally occurring groups in cities like San Francisco, where there is a relatively steady influx of Latino immigrants from Mexico, Central and South America, and the Caribbean, as well as a substantial number of U.S.-born Hispanics of Mexican descent (Chicanos). I would like to propose that several groups of Latino gay men who share important similarities and interact quite frequently can be described along a dimension of acculturation to the mainstream English-speaking culture or, more specifically, according to their level of integration and participation in the mainstream non-Hispanic White gay culture. Research along with clinical and personal observations by myself and others have indicated the existence of three distinct groups of self-identified Latino gay men: acculturated, non-acculturated, and bicultural.

Acculturated Men

This group of men are highly identified with and integrated to the non-Hispanic White gay culture and seldom participate in the affairs of the Latino community. Because their increased integration to the mainstream culture is done at the expense of their participation in the Latino community, their acculturation can be considered "transitional" or "subtractive," that is, a process of acculturation that is based on some degree of rejection of the culture of origin. Typically, this type of acculturation is motivated by experiences of homophobic abuse and rejection in the context of the Latino community or country of origin and a failure to successfully come out in the context of their native culture.

Thus acculturated men tend to feel "more gay than Latino" and have been able to identify themselves openly as gay mostly or exclusively in the context of the mainstream gay culture, perhaps at the expense of their Latino cultural identity. In fact, many of these men came to the U.S., or to places like San Francisco, in order to come out within the cultural context of the U.S. gay liberation movement and remove themselves from the pressures of immediate and close interactions with their homophobic families. Even if they were born in the U.S., acculturated men tend to denounce the homophobia of their native Latino communities and acknowledge the difficulties of coming out and living a life of authenticity among their Latino families. These men seldom go to

Latino-identified gay bars and instead prefer to socialize and participate in social, cultural, and political activities as non-ethnically defined
members of the mainstream gay community.

It is important to note that, in the context of this chapter, acculturation refers to Latino men's identification and participation within the
gay mainstream culture. As suggested by recent studies of acculturation
and biculturalism, such cultural participation must take into account
both competent skills and positive affect (LaFramboise et al. ., 1993;
Padilla, 1980). Many Latino gay men may be quite competent in dealing and functioning within the mainstream gay culture, but affectively
and emotionally they feel quite disconnected and ill-at-ease within it
for a number of different reasons, ranging from non-standard physical
appearance to institutionalized class and race discrimination practices
within the gay community.

The question still remains as to the actual or relative degree of acculturation possible for the (so-called) acculturated Latino gay men.
These men may be trying to escape the Latino homophobia through
rejection of their culture of origin and adopting a non-ethnically
defined gay culture which might, after all, not exist. In addition, it must
be recognized that these men were socialized as Latinos and may
remain at a very deep level "hopelessly Latinos," especially within the
domain of sexuality. It seems obvious that labeling this group of men as
"acculturated" must be done with a great deal of caution, in light of the
present scarcity of data about the processes of acculturation, language
use, and interactions with families and the gay community for this
group of men.

Non-Acculturated Men

On the other side of the acculturation continuum is a group of men
who are highly identified as Latinos, who prefer (or are only able) to
use the Spanish language among family and friends, and who socialize
in the context of Latino-identified groups, bars, and establishments.
Much of their gay life and sexuality center on traditional Latino sex
roles for homosexuals in Latin American countries, specifically the
sharp distinctions between feminine and masculine roles and prefer-
ences, where being gay is defined in terms of gender identity (a man
who feels and loves like a woman) rather than in terms of same-gender

sexual orientation (men who love men or who experience same-sex desire). Some in this group, however, do identify as gay men and are genuinely struggling to achieve and maintain a gay identity as men who love men, beyond the confines of rigidly defined sex roles in the Latino community.

In San Francisco, for example, three major groupings exist within the non-acculturated community with the following three recognizable but somewhat disparaging labels in parenthesis: feminine-identified *(Queenas)*, gay-identified *(Buchonas)*, and heterosexual-identified *(Bugarrones/Mayates)*. The first group is constituted by men who strongly identify with feminine sex and gender roles. Many of them cross-dress and move toward feminization through the intake of hormones and surgical procedures. These men do feel like "a woman in a man's body," have definite interests in beauty and fashion that are consistent with traditional female roles, and prefer heterosexual or straight-identified men as sexual partners since for many of them being homosexual means being a "woman" and they are attracted to "real" (i.e., straight) men.

It is for this reason perhaps that feminine-identified men refer to gay-identified homosexuals as *Buchonas*. The label *Buchona* cleverly combines the label "butch" for masculine-identified characteristics in the gay and lesbian communities with the Spanish feminine ending "-a," which somehow neutralizes the macho effect. It is my impression that feminine-identified men use the label *Buchona* to support their own definition of homosexuality as women inside men's bodies, suggesting that Latino gay-identified males who feel and act masculine simply haven't caught on to the idea that they are truly women. This is particularly true when referring to gay men who enjoy the receptive or passive role in anal sex. In one of the focus groups I conducted, when talking about a gay man who enjoyed receptive anal intercourse, a feminine-identified man said, *"Y ésa qué se cree? Ella es mujer"* ("And that one, who does she think she is? She is a woman").

It is important to note that, even for gay-identified males *(Buchonas)* in the non-acculturated group, the adherence and identification with society's definition of gender and gender roles may serve as important social and psychological organizers. The sharp distinctions between those who play the passive versus the active role in sexual intercourse and the meaning and impact such roles may have on their masculinity or "macho image" is a matter of concern, as well as a frequent subject of conversations and jokes. For example, the idea that a gay man is not a real man but someone who has *una loca* inside is quite prevalent in this group. When talking about a man that tried to appear virile but moved his hands in an effeminate way, several gay-identified men said, *"se le salió la loca!"* (his queen came out!). There is also the shared idea that gay men who want to be "active/inserters" and look masculine must work really hard at it—as if keeping the *loca* inside is quite an effortful and energy-consuming enterprise. If a gay man wants to put down another gay man, reference to *esa loca* (that queen) is quite effective, and occurs quite frequently I might add.

These observations underscore the fact that the Latino concept of homosexuality as some kind of psychological transgenderism, discussed in detail in Chapter 4, is more evident in non-acculturated gay men. However, as men in this group come in contact with the concepts and ideology of gay liberation movements both in the U.S. and Latin America, there seems to be an increased acceptance of versatility in taking active and receptive roles in sexual relations and an increased assurance in the possible integration and compatibility of masculinity and homosexuality. This is especially true of Latin American men who have migrated to this country after some activism within gay liberation movements in their own countries.

A third group of players in the world of non-acculturated Latino gay men is a group of heterosexual-identified men who like to have sex with men; they are derrogatively referred to as *Bugarrones* or *Mayates*, and it would be a mistake to consider them "homosexual" or "gay," as we currently define the terms. I believe that these heterosexual-identified men who have sex with other men should be studied on their own accord. However, no picture of the non-acculturated Latino gay community would be complete without reference to this important set of players.

It is widely acknowledged that many men in Latino cultures have sex with other men with no direct questioning of or impact on their self-identification as heterosexuals. This is especially true if they take the insertive or active role in anal intercourse and if their partners are effeminate or feminine-identified. In fact, for this group of men, the penetration of another man conveys feelings of power, strength, and masculinity that reinforces their heterosexual, macho identity. This phenomenon of homosexually reinforced heterosexuality can be understood in the context of a society that defines homosexuality in terms of gender rather than same-sex desires and behavior, and where masculinity must be prove by sexual penetration. For many Latino males, having another male "turn around and let you have him" would not be considered an insult but rather a sign of their strength, dominance, and masculinity, and ultimately flattering to the internalized macho ideal.

At this point, I feel compelled to insist that the labels used for the different members of the non-acculturated group in San Francisco, *Queenas, Buchonas,* and *Bugarrones/Mayates,* although informative on their own terms, can be highly deprecatory and insulting to the members of their respective groups. I have used these labels, somewhat reluctantly, because the labels themselves provide important windows of understanding to the culture of non-acculturated Latino men who engage in homosexual behavior. However, as social scientists we must be careful with the possible impact of labeling populations of interest with terms that can be derogatory and offensive. It is for this reason that these three groups of men should be referred to as feminine-identified, gay-identified, and heterosexual-identified. Moreover, these more appropriate labels can help us see that what is typically considered gay-identification in Western cultures—the adoption of same-sex desire and behavior as a focal point of self and social sexual identity—does not necessarily apply to many Latino men who engage in homosexual behavior.

Bicultural Men

There is an increasing number of Latino men who identify (or are in the process of identifying) as gay in both the Latino and mainstream gay cultures. These men frequently interact with other gay-identified Latinos and tend to choose one another as sexual and romantic partners. They are able to participate with varying degrees of comfort in mainstream gay activities, and some of them choose non-Latino gay men as their partners. They also tend to be active in Latino gay organizations, striving to support their dual cultural identification through organizational affiliation. They are the activists and community organizers who openly wage the dual battles against homophobia in the Latino community and racism and classism in the predominantly

White gay community. These men successfully incorporate, or are in the process of incorporating, the elements of both their gay and Latino identities.

The most important point that must be understood about bicultural Latino gay men can be stated as follows: Their gay identification is more similar to the mainstream gay culture rather than to the traditional roles for homosexuals in Latino communities. Therefore, these men tend to feel uncomfortable, and many times angry, with the Latino definitions of homosexuality and the rigidity of sex-role identification discussed above (similar to their more acculturated peers). On the other hand, the bicultural men's strong and militant identification as Latinos does not allow for a full identification or integration within what is considered to be a predominantly White, oppressive, and racist gay culture. These men are caught, so to speak, between a homophobic rock and a racist hard place.

Biculturalism, defined as competent and joyful participation in two different cultures, is a difficult process and goal to achieve. Thus the question needs to be raised whether bicultural Latino gay men do indeed participate successfully in two cultures, or rather feel alien and disconnected from both. I am afraid I cannot provide an answer to such an important question at this time. We need more empirical and in-depth studies in order to fully understand the processes involved in gay biculturalism and to uncover the processes by which men may actually achieve it with some degree of success.

These observations underscore the crucial importance of social support through Latino gay organizations and other militant groups for gay men in the process of becoming bicultural. While these men share the hope of integration, they also face the risk of disconnection and isolation from both cultures.

In Summary

It is important to note that the process of acculturation can be either additive or subtractive, depending on whether the individual in question moves toward integration (additive) or rejection (subtractive) of the culture of origin; the ultimate product of *additive* acculturation is genuine biculturalism. As such, acculturation refers to a set of complex psychosocial processes within individuals rather than to a demographic characteristic of groups. Even though, mostly for heuristic purposes, I have described groups of Latino gay men according to their accultura tion levels, the groups contain a great deal of individual variation in the processes of acculturation and integration of Latino and gay cultures. The boundaries between the groups are fuzzy and overlapping, rather than rigidly defined or mutually exclusive.

Nevertheless, I would like to argue that how individuals solve the integration between their Latino and gay identities, and at what stage of this process they are at a given time, will determine to a great extent who they interact with, what groups they will join, and how they will live and express their homosexual desires. The notion of acculturation groups is, therefore, a valid approach to understand and classify natu-rally occurring groups in this population. No clear or accurate under-standing of Latino gay men in the U.S. will be possible until we study individual variability in the processes of both subtractive and additive acculturation to the gay mainstream culture.

8.

A Psycho-Cultural Model of Sexual Self-Regulation

As a group and in comparison to other groups at risk, Latino gay men have relatively strong intentions to practice safer sex but concurrently a very high rate of risky sexual behavior. An over-arching goal of the present book is to search for an explanation of this apparent and puzzling incongruence between behavioral intentions and actual sexual behavior. This search has paved the way for a "psycho-cultural" theoretical framework or model that I believe can help us understand how cultural factors functionally compete with and against the enactment of safer sex intentions. In previous chapters, I have specified and elaborated the specific cognitive-cultural scripts that regulate the sexual activity of Latino gay men. In this chapter, I want to explore how, in the face of competing circumstances, volitional processes may break down and personal intentions to act safely may be discarded in a surrender of the "executive" self-regulatory self to more scripted, unconscious, and emotionally loaded psychological processes.

The label psycho-cultural underscores the fact that, in human development, cultural values that give guidance and provide structure to social relations among members of the culture become *internalized*, giving shape to individuals' construction of their sense of self and of their role in the social, interpersonal world including, of course, their values, perceptions, and meaning regarding sexuality. Cultural guidelines and proscriptions that regulate the behavior of individual members of the culture (such as what constitutes appropriate and valued male sexual behavior) become transferred or internalized as personal values, mores, and cognitive scripts that become the main regulators of individual behavior. In line with current sociocultural perspectives of human development, the model assumes that *inter*-personal (social) guidelines become internalized as *intra*-personal (psychological) regulators (Díaz, Neal, and Amaya-Williams, 1990).

The model addresses the possibility that, in the face of strong personal and interpersonal pressures against condom use, there might be a breakdown of intentional and volitional processes in the sexual activity of Latino gay men. I use the term *volition breakdown* to underscore the fact that, in the face of difficult and competing circumstances, personal intentions are not only weakened but may actually be discarded altogether, and not necessarily replaced by alternate personal intentions. I want to propose that at moments of volition breakdown, behavior is no longer guided by self-regulatory, intentional, "executive" processes, but rather it is guided and regulated by highly automatized, routinized, and mostly unconscious cognitive and cultural scripts. While the notion that sexual activity is guided and regulated by a set of culturally determined cognitive scripts is not new (see for example Gagnon and Simon, 1973), the notion that those scripts take over regulatory power in the face of a breakdown of intentional and volitional processes is a major claim of the psycho-cultural model proposed in this chapter.

Assumptions of the Psycho-cultural Model

The psycho-cultural model does not focus on variables and processes that lead to the formulation of safer sex intentions. Rather, in agreement with existing data for Latino gay men, the model assumes that there is in place a relatively strong behavioral intention to practice safer sex. The psycho-cultural model does recognize, however, that the failure to enact behavioral intentions will eventually affect the formulation and strength of future intentions—for example, by decreasing the sense of personal control and self-efficacy or by promoting a sense of personal helplessness and fatalism about the behavior in question. Thus, the model is compatible, to some extent, with social-learning formulations of self-regulation, such as Bandura's (1994) current conceptualizations of perceived self-efficacy in the practice of safer sex.

Unlike social-cognitive models, however, the psycho-cultural perspective proposes that, in the face of weakened personal intentions or a breakdown of intentionality, individuals' behaviors will be guided and regulated by internalized cultural factors, that is, cultural guidelines of behavior that are highly over-learned, routinized, scripted, and automatized. For the most part, individuals are not likely to be consciously aware of such cultural determinants of their individual behavior, and in response to questions about what happened in a given instance of risky behavior, they may simply and genuinely answer "I don't know."

A major tenet of this psycho-cultural perspective is that, because culture becomes internalized (culture becomes psychological, so to speak), it can exercise a great deal of influence on individuals in the relative absence of external guidance, support, and cultural reward systems. By *internalized* cultural factors, I mean that cultural scripts can be found not only in the social discourse *between* individuals but also in the cognitive schemata, values, and perceptions *within* individual members of the culture. The search for "psycho-cultural variables" in the domain of sexuality, therefore, becomes a search for the ways in which culture has become internalized and is now manifested in the individual's sexual attitudes, perceptions, and actual behavior.

Even though individuals' behavioral intentions are more easily enacted when these are congruent and supported by both the sociocultural context and the internalized cultural guidelines, it is true that many individuals can exercise a high degree of self-direction and self-determination over and above cultural, contextual, and situational determinants. That is why it is possible for many Latino men to enact safer sex intentions that seem to contradict internalized cultural norms and beliefs about masculinity such as "men cannot control their sexual impulses" or "losing your erection during sex is the most embarrassing thing." However, the central point is that those cultural constructions of what constitutes valued male behavior, for example, make the enactment of safer sex intentions much more difficult and perhaps close to impossible for those men whose sense of self-regulation and self-determination within the domain of sexuality is not particularly well developed. More important, those cultural scripts (among others) become the main regulators of behavior in the presence of a self-regulatory or volition breakdown in the practice of safer sex.

In summary, the psycho-cultural framework presented in this book rests on three central assumptions:

1. The first assumption is that sociocultural factors are not external to the individual members of the culture but rather have become internalized as cognitive scripts that guide and give personal meaning to sexual behavior.

2. Second, individuals have the capability to intend and perform new types of health-promoting behavior (such as condom use) in an executive, self-regulatory fashion, even if such behavior is at odds with cultural scripts or not particularly supported or reinforced by the immediate sociocultural context. However, the successful enactment of those intentions will depend on the strength of the individual's intention, the individual's capacity to exercise self-regulation and self-determination in the specific domain (e.g., sexuality), and the level of support—or conversely, the presence of competing variables—that exist in the immediate personal or interpersonal situation.

3. Third, the model assumes that in the face of difficult and challenging situations, there can be a breakdown in self-regulatory, volitional processes. In moments of volitional breakdown, cultural, cognitive, and sexual scripts, rather than self-formulated plans of action or personal intentions to engage in health-promoting behavior, will become the main regulators and determinants of sexual activity.

The psycho-cultural model of HIV risk has been developed to address and integrate the impact of both cultural regulation and self-regulation in the practice of safer sex. It is important, therefore, to visit both constructs of culture and self-regulation as conceptual foundations for the proposed model. In addition, because the model assumes that culture is internalized, it is important to examine with some detail the construct of internalization.

Cultural Theory

As a developmental psychologist who is an enthusiastic (though limited) consumer of anthropological literature, I am always pleasantly surprised at how "psychological" and how "developmental" are anthropologists' definition of culture. For example, when defining the concept of culture, medical anthropologist Cecil Helman (1990) visited both classical (Tylor, 1871) and contemporary (Keesing, 1981) attempts at defining this elusive concept. Helman concludes: ". . . culture is a set of guidelines (explicit and implicit) which individuals inherit as members of a particular society, and which tells them how to view the world, how to experience it *emotionally*, and how to *behave* in it . . . culture can be seen as an inherited 'lens,' through which individuals perceive and understand the world that they inhabit and learn how to live within it" (pp. 2–3). Because psychologists are interested in explaining human perception, emotions, and behavior, Helman's definition situates culture at the very heart of psychology's domain.

By providing the "guidelines" for perceptions, emotions, and behavior, culture can be understood as the main, socially shared regulator of cognitive, affective activity. Nowhere are these cultural guidelines more powerful and explicit than in the domain of gender and sexuality, that is, the domain of interest for the prevention of HIV in Latino gay men. The majority of cultural groups have explicit guidelines about what constitutes appropriate, valued, and forbidden behavior in sexual communication, extramarital sex, and homosexual activity. Because these guidelines are typically specified in relation to what is valued and appropriate for the two different genders, they become internalized as part of a strongly reinforced and deeply ingrained gender socialization process.

Helman's definition of culture is also elaborated along a truly developmental dimension: "Growing up within any society is a form of *en*culturation, whereby the individual slowly acquires the cultural 'lens' of that society" (p. 3). In development, gender-related sexual guidelines, the *social* gender, become an integral part of what is labeled by Helman (1990) the *psychological* gender, that is, individuals' gender self-definition in terms of self-perception and sexual behavior. Thus, for most socialized members of the human species, culturally given guidelines for gender-appropriate sexual behavior become the principal lens through which individuals perceive, feel, and act their own sexuality.

When current conceptualizations of culture and enculturation are taken into account, the label *psycho*-cultural seems a bit redundant; the label "cultural" would have sufficed. However, I have decided to keep the label psycho-cultural, especially for those individuals (in particular, psychologists) who still conceptualize culture as outside the domain of psychology, for those who still see culture as outside the individual.

Even though there are some excellent proposals in the field of developmental psychology to develop a truly cultural psychology, mostly inspired by the work of Vygotsky and cognitive approaches to anthropology (see, for example, Stigler et al., 1990), with few exceptions, these proposals have not yet reached those interested in theories of health psychology and behavior change in the field of HIV prevention research.

Self-Regulation

The psycho-cultural model of HIV risk proposed and developed in the present paper is a theoretical framework to help us understand problems in the self-regulation of sexuality. More specifically, the model is being developed to understand the hypothesized breakdown of self-regulatory or volitional functioning in the domain of sexuality among Latino gay men. It is of paramount importance, therefore, to define and discuss the construct of self-regulation, as it is understood in the work of psychology today.

Self-regulation can be formally defined as the human capacity to plan, guide, and monitor one's behavior flexibly in the face of difficult and challenging circumstances (see Díaz, 1990, 1991). In self-regulation, the sources of behavioral control are to be found not in the immediate and external environmental stimuli, but rather in an *internal and self-generated cognitive plan or behavioral intention* that has been formulated by an individual to achieve desirable goals. Thus, when individuals are functioning in a self-regulated manner, the behavior of such individuals is guided or regulated not by contingencies (punishment and rewards) found in the immediate environment, but by a self-generated plan or behavioral intention that might be quite independent from immediate consequences (expected, imagined, and actual). It is important to remember that many health-promoting behaviors involve immediate personal sacrifices for the sake of long-term positive outcomes and, as such, health-promoting behaviors more often than not demand and assume a great deal of self-regulatory capacity and self-regulated level of functioning.

For developmental psychologists, self-regulation refers to the person's decreasing dependence on external, social, and caregiving structures, and the increasing reliance on self-formulated goals, plans, and intentions for the regulation of behavior. Self-regulation is also considered a developmental pathway, a movement from other-regulation to self-regulation, signaling children's increasing autonomous functioning from caregivers' dictates and supportive external structures. Thus, in developmental psychology, self-regulation is considered to be not a set of learned skills but rather a "property" or "quality" of human activity— a level of "functional organization" achieved in development.

Bandura (1986), from a somewhat different perspective, has eloquently written about this quality of human behavior as the capacity for self-direction:

> If actions were determined solely by external rewards and punishments, people would behave like weathervanes, constantly shifting direction to conform to whatever momentary influence happened to impinge upon them. They would act corruptly with unprincipled people and honorably with right-principled ones, and liberally with libertarians and dogmatically with authoritarians. In actuality, *except when subjected to coercive pressure*, people display considerable self-direction in the face of many competing influences. (p. 335, emphasis mine)

In Bandura's social cognitive perspective, self-regulation involves the enactment of three interrelated but distinct and sequentially ordered subprocesses (also labeled subfunctions): self-observation, judgmental process, and self-reaction. In his own words, "Self-regulation is not achieved by a feat of willpower. It operates through a set of subfunctions that must be developed and mobilized for self-directed change" (1986, p. 336). *Self-observation* refers to individuals' abilities to observe and understand the causes and determinants of their own behavior, including the personal, contextual, and situational factors that influence their psychological functioning and sense of well-being. Once personal behavior has been observed, individuals must be able to evaluate it, favorably or negatively, in light of a set of internal standards. The processes involved in this evaluative judgment of personal behavior are labeled the *judgmental subfunction*. Finally, as suggested by the third and last subcomponent, *self-reaction*, individuals must be able to react or respond actively to their judgmental processes, mostly by creating conditions that motivate desired behavior and decrease undesirable ones. According to Bandura, by creating personal incentives—contingent rewards or self-motivators that reinforce valued behavior—individuals manipulate strategically their own person-situation context to facilitate the enactment of difficult intentions.

As Bandura's exception ("when subjected to coercive pressure") suggests, self-regulation is limited and, as a level of functioning, can break down in certain coercive circumstances. It is my belief, however, that *external* coercion (such as peer pressure) is only *one* of the possible competing circumstances that may contribute to a breakdown of self-direction or self-regulation. For example, deep emotions originated and subjectively experienced within the person, such as an overwhelming desire for flesh-to-flesh contact or an extreme fear of embarrassment and rejection, might strongly compete with the enactment of safer sex intentions and pose difficulties similar to external coercion.

Acknowledging that individuals' intentions often must be enacted in the face of competing circumstances, German psychologists Julius Kuhl and Jurgen Beckmann (1985) have defined self-regulation in terms of protecting an intention from what they label *competing action tendencies*, that is, from those factors that compete with and undermine its enactment. Somewhat differently from Bandura, Kuhl and Beckmann define self-regulation as within the domain of volition, that is, the domain of psychology that, in contrast to cognition and motivation, is particularly concerned with intention-behavior relations. Self-regulation is thus defined as the set of processes that protects and maintains the intention until enactment has been successfully completed.

> Despite the continuous pressure exerted by competing action tendencies, people often stick to the behavioral intention they are currently committed to until the goal is reached. This phenomenon suggests the existence of processes that prevent competing tendencies from becoming dominant before the current goal is reached. . . . The terms *volitional control*, *action control*, and *self-regulation* will be used here interchangeably to denote those processes which *protect* a current intention from being replaced should one of the competing tendencies increase in strength before the intended action is completed. (Kuhl and Beckmann, 1985, p. 102)

Kuhl and Beckmann's theory of action control defines self-regulation as precisely the processes by which intentions are enacted. Central to the enactment of intentions are individuals' actual attempts at protecting their intentions from competing action tendencies. In line with Bandura's theorizing, they suggest that self-regulation is characterized by individuals' implementation of strategies that modify internal processes (e.g., a shift of attentional focus) as well as situational and contextual variables (e.g., avoiding persons and circumstances that create social pressure) in ways that would favor and support the enactment of the particular intention until the personal goal is successfully achieved.

Because the capacity for self-direction or self-regulation is an outcome of human development, we should expect individual differences in the ability to self-regulate and exercise self-direction in the face of competing circumstances. However, as both Bandura's and Kuhl and Beckmann's theories suggest, self-regulated functioning (i.e., actual self-regulated or self-directed behavior) cannot be understood simply as a property of the individual. Even though self-regulatory functioning assumes the individual's capacity to act beyond (or in spite of) immediate environmental contingencies, paradoxically, self-regulatory functioning is made possible—either enhanced or seriously limited—by the properties of the context in which it occurs. In other words, individuals' actual expression of self-regulation in a given situation can be either supported or severely limited by the number and strength of competing variables that exist in the particular person-situation context.

I would like to propose that there might be a complex and compensatory relationship between the strength of an individual's capacity for self-regulation on the one hand, and the strength of the competing factors on the other where, in order for self-regulated behavior (i.e., the enactment of personal intentions) to occur, the individual's self-regulatory strength and effort must be greater than the strength of the competing variables. In other words, the amount of self-regulatory effort that is demanded in a given situation is directly a function of the strength of the competing variables. It follows that, in the relative absence of competing variables, the majority of individuals will be able to enact their intentions with little self-regulatory effort, but in the face of extremely difficult circumstances, only those with a really strong self-regulatory capacity might be able to maintain, protect, and enact their intentions.

Two important questions emerge from this discussion: How can we define self-regulatory strength and effort? And more important, how can we promote it? In light of current theories of self-regulation, I would like to propose that self-regulatory strength is constituted by two important psychological functions: (1) the individual's capacity for self-observation and awareness of competing factors in the enactment of a given intention, and (2) the individual's repertoire of actively constructed strategies and shills to modify the person-situation context in ways congruent with the intention.

It is my belief that accurate self-observation and effective strategic modification of the person-situation context to protect the enactment of an intention is most likely domain-specific. For example, someone might be a keen self-observer and quite an agent of change in the domain of business transactions or in the domain defined by academic success; however, those self-regulatory abilities might not transfer simply when the domain in question is the person's own sexual behavior. In addition, I believe that self-observation and self-directed modification of the person-situation context are not necessarily skills that can be learned through training, but rather they are psychological functions that must be developed and co-constructed in social collaboration with other members of the community.

Chapter 9 will present a model of an HIV risk reduction intervention designed to promote sexual self-regulation. The program, entitled *Hermanos de Luna y Sol* (Brothers of Moon and Sun), targets Spanish-speaking, mostly immigrant, Latino gay and bisexual men in San Francisco. In the context of this program, I have had the opportunity to facilitate the processes of self-observation and strategy construction for the practice of safer sex. I will describe the program in detail as one particular example of an intervention that was designed and is being implemented guided by the findings and theory presented in this book.

Internalization

The increasing autonomy that individuals display in development is achieved not simply by a separation or moving away from external sources of regulation, but rather by a transferral of the sources of regulation from the inter-personal to the intra-personal domains, from the social to the psychological. This transference or movement from external (social) to internal (personal) sources of regulation is labeled "internalization."

It should be noted, however, that such internalization is not a mere passive transfer of values from the social culture to the individual, but rather involves an active co-construction of values and meaning by the individual in social discourse and collaboration with more expert members of the culture. This active co-construction of cultural guidelines reinforces individuals' perceptions that those guidelines are their own and, in a deep sense, they are because they have been actively co-constructed by individuals with the assistance of more expert members of the culture. When socialization and internalization processes have been successful and effective, cultural guidelines of behavior are subjectively experienced as one's own, as coming from within, with a great deal of personal conviction and commitment. This is particularly obvious in many Latino men's elaborate statements, typically expressed with great conviction and personal commitment, of what they believe is "manly" behavior.

It is important to realize, however, that the development of self-regulation cannot be described solely as the internalization of social and cultural mores. The development of self-regulation involves the emergence of an "executive" self that must be explained beyond the mere internalization of social and cultural guidelines of behavior. In fact, concurrent with this process of internalization, there emerges a sense of self—an emerging voice of self-regulation and self-determination—that evolves as distinct and unique with respect to other members of the social group. While different cultural groups and different individuals within those groups vary in the salience and strength of their separate sense of self and their capacity for self-determination, it is clear that for the majority of individuals a sense of self and self-determination does indeed emerge in development. Furthermore, such a personal self is capable of formulating and enacting behavioral intentions that could be quite at odds with cultural norms and guidelines of behavior; hence the concepts of *self*-regulation and *self*-determination, in contrast to being guided, regulated, or controlled by others in the social environment.

Outline for a Psycho-Cultural Model of HIV Risk

In outline form, the psycho-cultural model of sexual self-regulation, with specific reference to the practice of safer sex to avoid HIV infection, can be stated in terms of the following ten propositions:

1. In development, cultural guidelines about gender-appropriate sexual behavior become internalized as personal beliefs and cognitive scripts for sexual activity.

2. Many of these cultural guidelines, beliefs, and scripts (e.g., men can't control their sexual impulses; non-penetrative sex is no sex at all) are at odds with guidelines for safer sex practices.

3. Individual members of different cultural groups, however, are able to formulate and enact safer sex intentions in a self-regulatory fashion, even when the intentions are not supported by their cultural guidelines and scripts or their immediate sociocultural context.

4. To the extent that safer sex intentions are in competition with cultural guidelines and scripts, individuals need to exercise a higher level of self-regulatory strength.

5. Self-regulatory capacity, defined as the ability for self-observation and strategy construction, is domain specific, limited, and varies across individuals.

6. In the face of strong competition, personal, interpersonal, or contextual, against safer sex intentions, there is a possible breakdown of intentional, volitional, self-regulatory functioning. This breakdown of intentionality in sexual activity cannot be simply described as the replacement of the original intention with another more congruent intention.

7. In the case of self-regulatory breakdown, internalized cultural guidelines and scripts take over the regulation of individual behavior, and quite often this occurs with no or limited self-awareness and a deeply felt sense of lack of control over one's sexual behavior.

8. Because at times of volition breakdown, sexual behavior is regulated by internalized cultural norms and cognitive scripts, "risky" behavior is subjectively experienced as *meaningful* behavior from the given sociocultural perspective, and it is not necessarily experienced as "risk taking."

9. Even though the psycho-cultural model assumes the presence of relatively strong personal intentions for safer sex, and individuals' initial attempts to enact them, as a result of frequent enactment failure, there is a weakening of perceptions of self-efficacy and self-control and the development of a certain helplessness and

fatalism that undermines the formulation and enactment of future intentions.

10. The volition breakdown postulated by the psycho-cultural model does *not* explain all instances of risky sexual practices. Some individuals, for different reasons, engage in unprotected sex with full awareness and intentionality. Some individuals also take calculated risks in the practice of safer sex with full awareness of possible negative consequences. The psycho-cultural model is best used to explain unsafe behavior that happens in the presence of individuals' intentions and personal commitments to practice safer sex. Typically, in these situations, individuals are not able to articulate or explain fully why risky behavior actually occurs and might be quite puzzled about why they are continuing to practice risky sex with the best and strongest intentions not to do so.

The psycho-cultural model of HIV risk builds on Bandura's and Kuhl and Beckmann's theories of self-regulation. On one hand, the psycho-cultural model recognizes from current theories that (a) self-regulated behavior can be best defined as a person-situation variable rather than solely the property of an individual, (b) self-regulatory capacity is based upon individuals' self-observations and conscious awareness of the causes and determinants of their own behavior, and (c) self-regulation is enacted by individuals' active manipulation or modification of competing factors in the person-situation context, in ways that facilitate the enactment of a given intention.

On the other hand, the psycho-cultural model expands and builds on current theories of self-regulation in three specific ways: (a) it suggests the possibility that weakened intentions are not simply replaced by stronger intentions but rather, in the face of strong competing factors, there might be a possible breakdown of volitional and intentional behavior; (b) the model further suggests that, in the face of a volition breakdown, behavior is no longer regulated by an individual's consciously formulated intention but rather by highly automatized, routinized, and internalized cultural guidelines of behavior; and (c) finally, the model underscores the fact that there is a compensatory relation between individuals' self-regulatory strength and competing circumstances, where a volition breakdown is less likely to occur in the case when an individual's self-regulatory capacity and effort is stronger than the factors that compete with the enactment of the given intention. In other words, little self-regulatory strength and effort will be required to enact an intention in situations where competing factors are minimal; this is why, in line with Kuhl and Beckman, we must assume that self-regulatory effort must be exercised only in the face of difficult and challenging circumstances.

After carefully listening to the voices and struggles of Latino gay men, including my own, I am convinced that the practice of safer sex is particularly difficult for us and, therefore, the successful enactment of safer sex intentions will demand a great deal of self-regulatory effort in our sexual activity. However, I want to argue that self-observation in the domain of sexuality—the major ingredient of sexual self-regulation—has been seriously limited for Latino gay men, considering our socialization in the context of strong homophobic attitudes and a socially imposed silence about our sexuality. Furthermore, I believe that the homophobia and sexual silence in our culture—in our families, churches, and communities—have promoted a virtual *dissociation* of sexuality from the interpersonal, rational, and affective lives of many of us who experience same-sex desire. Such dissociation is perhaps the major obstacle to sexual self-regulation for Latino gay men, because the psychosocial construction of homosexuality as the domain of the secret, the forbidden, and the shameful has made self-observation in this domain extremely difficult and loaded with deeply felt but poorly understood emotions.

In the context of strong competing factors, and in the presence of a limited ability to self-regulate sexual activity, it is no surprise that Latino gay men constitute one of the most vulnerable groups in the nation for the transmission of HIV. Limitations in the ability to self-regulate sexuality, however, should not be understood as the result of a personal deficit, but rather as the natural outcome of socialization within a culture that promotes sexual silence about homosexual activity; splits off sexuality from the interpersonal, affective, and rational lives of gay men at the same time that it undermines perceptions of sexual control; and breeds fatalism. The causes for the sexual self-regulatory problems observed in Latino gay men can be found within the context of our socialization into a homophobic-machista culture, coupled with harsh experiences of poverty and racism as members of an ethnic minority group in the U.S.

9.

Hermanos de Luna y Sol

A Model for HIV Prevention
with Latino Gay Men

Throughout this book, I have offered a cultural analysis of risky sexual practices among Latino gay men, underscoring the fact that sociocultural factors, rather than personal intentions, are the major regulators of sexual behavior. As a Latino gay man who lives in a community highly affected by HIV, I must state as firmly as possible that *we do not have the time to wait* for major societal and cultural changes in order to promote behavior change and implement aggressive HIV prevention programs. The proposed psycho-cultural model of HIV risk (Chapter 8) emphasizes not only cultural factors but also their internalization and impact on individuals' sexual lives. Therefore, we must address not only the cultural sources of oppression but also their impact on individual men within specific subgroups in the population. If nothing else, we are called to promote sexual self-regulation in those who are most at risk.

My qualitative research to date suggests that sexual self-regulation among Latino gay men is jeopardized by a host of complex sociocultural factors, including machismo, homophobia, sexual silence, family loyalty, poverty, and racism, all of which contribute to (a) decreased self-esteem, (b) perceptions of low sexual control, (c) a sense of social isolation, and (d) fatalism regarding the inevitability of HIV infection. The situation is further complicated by the frequent use of drugs and alcohol during sex, multiple anonymous encounters in public sex environments, and situations of financial dependence leading to prostitution and sexual relations with men of unequal power and status.

In collaboration with Latino gay men who are health educators in San Francisco's Mission Neighborhood Health Center, we designed a program, *Hermanos de Luna y Sol* (HLS), to affect and modify these important predictors of risky sexual behavior. We were guided by the assumption that, in the midst of the six fold oppressive context, prevention efforts could be oriented to facilitate communication, self-observation, and critical reflection about these forces that regulate our sexuality. In addition, we believed that prevention programs could collaborate with the construction of personal strategies to deal effectively with barriers to safer sex practices created by the six sociocultural factors in the experiences of individual men. The program was originally funded by the Centers for Disease Control and Prevention (CDC) and, beginning in March 1997, its implementation continues with a three-year grant from the San Francisco Department of Health, AIDS Office.

After carefully reviewing both the quantitative and qualitative data on Latino gay men, we concluded that prevention programs could be effective if they: (1) break the sexual silence by providing safe venues for serious *communication about our sexuality*; (2) provide an *experience of communality and pride*, where men can feel part of a supportive and proud Latino gay community; (3) provide *opportunities for critical self-reflection and self-observation* about the factors that regulate our sexual behavior; (4) collaborate in the *construction of group, dyadic, and individual strategies* to address the perceived barriers to safer sex; and (5) create *opportunities for social activism* against the sociocultural and socioeconomic forces that undermine our self-determination and sexual self-regulation.

Thus, the overall goal of the intervention is to reduce the episodes of risky sexual behavior by increasing individuals' abilities to address and modify the person-situation factors that undermine or compete with the enactment of safer sex intentions. Based on the psycho-cultural model of HIV risk, Bandura's theory of self-regulation, and principles of empowerment education, HLS aims to intervene in a culturally appropriate manner with factors that weaken the enactment of safer sex intentions. By providing opportunities for group reflection and critical self-observation within the domain of sexuality, by providing peer social support for the practice of safer sex, and by sponsoring activities that support self-esteem and pride for being Latino and gay, the program intervenes with and attempts to modify factors that promote HIV risk behavior in this particular population.

As detailed below, the HLS program consists of three types of interrelated interventions: (1) bar outreach and recruitment activities; (2) four-meeting cycles with structured sessions designed to promote self-esteem, social support, and sexual self-regulation; and (3) a set of follow-up resources and activities targeted to the maintenance of safer sex behavior over time, including a safer sex journal, participation in an ongoing peer-support group, and access to prevention case-management services. The intervention was designed to target mostly immigrant, Spanish-speaking, gay men of low socioeconomic status in San Francisco's Mission District.

Theoretical Framework

The development of the intervention was guided by the integration of three conceptual frames: (1) Bandura's theory of self-regulation; (2) principles of empowerment education; and (3) the psycho-cultural model of HIV risk, as applied to the specific situation of Latino gay and bisexual men.

Bandura's Theory of Self-Regulation

In Bandura's (1986) social cognitive perspective, discussed in more detail in Chapter 8, self-regulation involves the enactment of three interrelated but distinct and sequentially ordered subprocesses (also labeled sub-functions): *self-observation, judgmental process,* and *self-reaction.* Based on accurate self-observation, self-regulation is characterized by individuals' implementations of strategies that modify both internal processes (e.g., a shift of attentional focus) and situational and contextual variables (e.g., avoiding persons and circumstances that create social pressure) in ways that would favor and support the enactment of a particular intention.

Bandura's theory of self-regulation was chosen for three specific reasons: (1) Qualitative studies suggest that the sexual behavior of Latino gay men is regulated by internalized, overlearned, and routinized cultural norms and patterns of behavior, and a great deal of unsafe behavior occurs without specific awareness of how those cultural determinants of behavior undermine the practice of safer sex. Thus, interventions aimed at behavior change in this population must start with the facilitation of sexual self-observation. (2) A review of the quantitative literature suggests that unsafe behavior occurs in the presence of relatively strong intentions to practice safe sex. Bandura's theory of self-regulation addresses the complex intention-behavior relation and processes by which intentions can be successfully enacted. (3) Finally, theories of self-regulation address the issue of relapse and the maintenance of safe sex behavior over time and across difficult situations; our intention was to develop an intervention that would provide the tools to maintain safer sex over time in the face of difficult and competing circumstances.

Principles of Empowerment Education

The method of empowerment education is used for promoting the functions of self-observation, evaluative judgments, and the development of self-reactive strategies. The most basic principle of empowerment pedagogy is that individuals and communities (rather than professionals) must define their own problems or difficulties and devise their own solutions (Freire, 1993). The professional or educator's role is thus to *facilitate* or *collaborate* with this process of self-defining problems and strategic solutions. This collaboration is achieved by asking challenging questions, by presenting "eye-opening" data or facts about the community, by promoting critical thinking about specific problems and potential courses of action to address them, and by mirroring, reflecting, and articulating the self-defined problems in order to elicit the construction of strategic courses of action (Shor, 1992). Because, in this model of education, strategic skills are self-constructed rather than externally given, empowerment methods were chosen as the most efficient way to promote self-regulatory functioning in the sexual domain.

Sociocultural Barriers to HIV Prevention in Latino Gay Men

The HLS intervention recognizes that risky sexual behavior does not happen as a result of a personal deficit in knowledge, motivation, or skills. Rather, the intervention takes into account that risky sex is meaningful behavior that is encouraged and promoted by the particular sociocultural context described in previous chapters. Therefore, when the program targets issues of self-esteem, social alienation, and fatalism, for example, it does so from the perspectives of the six sociocultural factors that have become competing barriers to the practice of safer sex. By contextualizing personal instances of unsafe behavior in culturally meaningful ways, we create a non-punitive discourse about individuals' risky sex and raise awareness about cultural regulators of individual sexual behavior.

Target Population

The program is specifically targeted to Latino men who attend Latino-identified gay bars in San Francisco's Mission District. Because we have chosen to target gay bar patrons, a definitely high-risk group, we provide services to men who self-identify as gay or bisexual in the Latino community, rather than the more inclusive men who have sex with men (MSM) category. However, many of our targeted self-identified gay and bisexual men are not publicly identified as such. Therefore, our interventions are sensitive to and take into account the specific difficulties of "coming out" for this group of men. Of special concern are issues related to coming out to families for whom a child's homosexuality is typically a source of shame and dishonor.

By targeting bar patrons of Latino-identified bars in San Francisco's Mission District, we are targeting Spanish-speaking, non-acculturated men, mostly of low socioeconomic status. Unlike Latinos who actively participate in the mainstream gay community, for example, non-acculturated men participate in a unique culture of homosexual behavior that is typical of rural Latin America and non-industrialized countries. Our interventions take into account unique aspects of this culture, such as the fact that homosexuality is defined as a gender rather than an orientation issue, homosexuals are seen as women in men's bodies or as less than "real" men, and a high prevalence of transvestite and transgender persons (hence the program name "of Moon and Sun," with implicit reference to the integration of masculine and feminine characteristics).

In addition, many non-acculturated men retain strong ties to their families and the straight Latino community, often at the price of silence about their lives and a sense of personal isolation and alienation.

This sense of isolation is reinforced by a lack of integration to the mainstream (mostly White) gay community due to issues of language, racism, and classism, and a lack of integration to workplace, church, or social organizations because of strong homophobia in the Latino community. Thus, a major goal of the intervention is to provide a sense of communality and consistent sources of social support.

Essential Elements of the Intervention

There are four essential experiences that we want HLS participants to have:

1. *An experience of group communality and safety.* Through the exploration of a common history, including experiences of homophobia, machismo, sexual abuse, and separation from family and country, the group must achieve first a distinctive sense of cohesion and bonding. This sense of communality is typically achieved by leading the group to discuss the question, "What is the most difficult thing about being a Latino gay man?"

Concurrent with the experience of social cohesiveness as members of an oppressed and victimized community, the group is defined as the place where we can "be ourselves," without fear of rejection or ridicule, where participants can "take off our protective masks" and be listened to and understood by others. Group rules regarding confidentiality, non-judgmental opinions, and mutual respect contribute to a definition of the group meetings as a safe place to communicate about intimate and personal matters.

2. *Awareness of the impact of AIDS on sexual activity.* A group discussion about the impact of HIV and AIDS in our lives, and specifically the impact of HIV on our sexual practices is, in our experience, the best way to introduce the topic of difficulties in the practice of safer sex. This discussion is motivated by the question, "How have you been affected by the AIDS epidemic?" This is followed up with questions about changes in sexual feelings and behavior in response to the epidemic. The discussion on the devastating impact of AIDS provides the context for Bandura's judgmental subfunction, where safer sex is established by the group as the only viable alternative for protection, health, and ultimate survival of the community.

3. *Critical thinking about barriers to safer sex.* A guided exploration of

those circumstances—personal, interpersonal, and situational—that make the practice of safer sex difficult is perhaps the most crucial aspect of the intervention. This discussion is prompted first by a general question, "What makes safer sex difficult for you?" This question is followed by more specific questions based on the sociocultural barriers to safer sex that were identified in the qualitative study of San Francisco gay men. At times, the group is asked to participate in activities where they can list elements of a difficult context or situation to practice safer sex. These and activities facilitate a highly focused and specifically targeted process of self-observation in the domain of safer sex practices.

In response to the question "What is the most difficult thing for you in the practice of safer sex?" men have been able to reflect on barriers and obstacles to their consistent condom use. For example, a major barrier articulated by many participants is the fact that the use of condoms makes them lose their erection. Further questioning, however, has led to a self-observation that the loss of erection is not so much a matter of physical sensations but rather a consequence of a learned association or connection between condoms and illness, death, and loss caused by the AIDS epidemic. Condoms bring up deep emotions of loss and grief, thus interfering with sexual arousal. Moreover, the loss of erection is extremely disturbing to many, as it undermines the erotic experience of masculine energy sought in same-sex encounters.

4. *Formulation of self-reactive strategies and skills.* A major goal of the group process is to help participants articulate and construct strategies in response to the stated difficulties, including the possibility of avoiding those difficulties that undermine their sense of personal control over sexual behavior. This goal (akin to Bandura's self-reaction) is achieved first by the facilitator's rephrasing the stated difficulties and asking participants, "If you were a counselor or a health educator, a brother or a friend, and someone told you they had this difficulty, what would you say?" This question allows participants to react to their stated difficulties in the context of more expert members of their peer group and use the group interactions to construct health-promoting strategies. The goal here is to facilitate the self-construction of strategic courses of action in response to self-defined problems in the practice of safer sex.

We typically mirror the stated barrier (e.g., fear of losing erection) to the group and direct them, "Imagine you are a counselor (or older brother) and one of your clients (or younger brother) has this problem ... what would you suggest?" The group then begins to construct and develop strategies to deal with this particular competing barrier—suggesting, for example, that they could move their attention away from the penis and focus on specific parts of their partners' bodies that have strong erotic charges for them (e.g., nipples, the back of the neck, muscular legs, etc.). In this example, participants came to the conclusion that they could recover their sexual arousal if they focused their attention on other "masculine," erotically charged aspects of themselves or their partners. Their strategy construction underscored the fact that focusing attention on the erection loss would only contribute to a further decrease of arousal.

Interestingly, Kuhl and Beckmann's action-control theory postulates that one of the most important self-regulatory strategies for the enactment of difficult intentions is "attention regulation," that is, the ability to shift attention away from the competing variable and focus on variables or factors that support it. In the example given, the men from *Hermanos de Luna y Sol* were spontaneously constructing a culturally appropriate and highly contextualized strategy of attention regulation in the domain of sexual activity.

The self-observation and strategy construction I have witnessed in the context of *Hermanos de Luna y Sol* have shown me that it is possible to promote sexual self-regulation as an effective tool for HIV prevention with Latino gay men. It is precisely these processes of self-observation and strategy construction that have been missing from many HIV-prevention programs that simply encourage condom use as a health guideline that must be complied with. In my opinion, those programs might promote compliance but not sexual self-regulation.

Intervention Components

Bar Outreach and Recruitment Activities

The bar outreach and recruitment program consists of a 5 to 10 minute survey, done at the bars, where Latino gay bar patrons are asked to answer eight questions. The surveys are administered by trained outreach workers in one-to-one conversations at the bars. The survey serves two major purposes: First, by asking bar patrons to reflect on issues related to HIV and AIDS and safer sex, the survey constitutes a brief outreach intervention to promote discussion and awareness of concerns related to HIV transmission and prevention. Second, the brief survey serves as advertisement and recruitment for the group interventions.

The survey questions cover some of the topics that are discussed in the program's group sessions. The outreach survey basically involves the experience of an informal, friendly, but serious, conversation about issues of concern to Latino gay men, including sexuality and HIV. Thus, the survey gives bar patrons a flavor of the kinds of topics and the kinds of discussions that can and will happen in the small group intervention.

The survey (administered in Spanish for the HLS target population) follows:

HI! I AM A MEMBER OF THE PROGRAM *HERMANOS DE LUNA Y SOL* AND WOULD LIKE TO TALK TO YOU FOR ABOUT FIVE MINUTES.

I WOULD LIKE TO ASK YOU SOME QUESTIONS THAT COULD HELP US HAVE A BETTER PROGRAM.

THIS INTERVIEW IS COMPLETELY ANONYMOUS AND CONFIDENTIAL; I DON'T NEED YOUR NAME.

1. How do you identify yourself with respect to sexual orientation?
2. Where, other than the bar, can you meet, talk, and have fun with other Latino gay men?
3. As a Latino gay man, what are you mostly concerned about?
4. Please tell me how important the following concerns are to you (to be rated on a 4-point scale of relative importance).

lovers and boyfriends	sexuality
family	work and profession
friendships	rejection of gay people
your health	social acceptance

5. Who can you talk to about these concerns on a regular basis?
6. On a scale of 1–10, how concerned are you about AIDS and HIV?
7. What is the most difficult thing for you about the practice of safer sex?
8. What has helped you the most to practice safer sex?

At the end of the interview, participants are given a ticket valid for a non-alcoholic drink at the bar, thanked for their participation in the survey, and given a card with the name, logo, and phone number of the program. They are told:

"We have organized a program that brings together Latino gay and bisexual men to discuss our most important concerns in a friendly and confidential small-group atmosphere. We get together in groups of 8 to 10 (with a facilitator who is also a Latino gay man) and have group discussions about some of the topics we just talked about. If you have questions about our program or are interested in coming to the groups, please call this number."

Men are enrolled in the program for the group meetings when they call the project number.

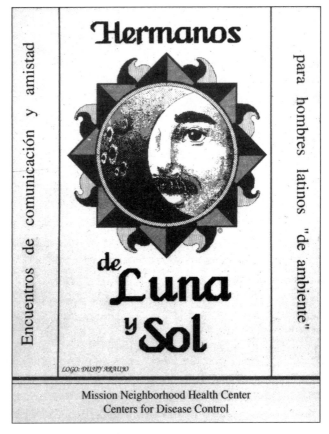

Figure 1. The outreach card for *Hermanos de Luna y Sol*. Text and graphic design by Rómulo Hernández.

The Outreach Card

The major and most frequent point of contact between the program and the target community is our outreach card (see Figure 1), masterfully created by Rómulo Hernández, HLS Project Coordinator. The card was designed very carefully in order to maximize our recruitment efforts; it is important, therefore, to examine it closely as a culturally appropriate tool to reach, motivate, and recruit members of the target population.

Note that unlike many HIV prevention materials distributed in the gay community, this card contains no sexually explicit images and makes no explicit or implicit reference to HIV (with the exception of

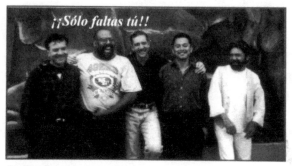

¡Te invitamos a descubrir qué tenemos en común!
La cena ya está servida y sólo falta que tú te incorpores a nuestras conversaciones.
Se trata de un nuevo programa para hombres "gay" y bi-sexuales latinos que consiste en 4 reuniones donde se intercambian opiniones sobre temas que a tí y a mí interesan.

¡¡Sólo faltas tú!!

Foto: Mary Schroeder

* Recibirás $10 por cada reunión y una franela (T-shirt) por tu asistencia a todo el ciclo.
🍴 Serviremos cena en cada reunión

Para mayor información e inscripción llama a Rómulo al 552-1013 Ext. 212

The back of the outreach card for *Hermanos de Luna y Sol*.

the fact that the names Mission Neighborhood Health Center, the sponsoring institution, and Centers for Disease Control, the funding agency, appear on the card). The program is presented as "encounters of friendship and communication for Latino men *de ambiente*" (*Encuentros de comunicacion y amistad para hombres de ambiente*). The card thus addresses directly two of the more important risk variables we want to target: sexual silence and social alienation. In response to those two risk factors, the program is offered as a place to connect in friendship with peers, and a place to speak out and communicate.

De ambiente (literally "of the environment" or "of the ambiance") is a popular Latino expression referring collectively to all those who are homosexually active or self-identify as homosexual, even though perhaps only privately so. Unlike many other collective labels for homosexuals, the phrase was formulated by homosexuals themselves and connotes no deprecating meaning. *De ambiente* is thus a code phrase that denotes (in-group) knowledge about sexual orientation and behavior, but does so in a private, self-referenced way, without the implication of being out publicly within a visible gay community. *De ambiente* was chosen for two major reasons: first, it places our program midway between society's silence about homosexuality, on the one hand, and forcing participants to identify as members of an open gay community on the other; and second, *de ambiente* is a more inclusive category than gay and bisexual, including homosexuals who do not identify as gay as well as transvestite and transgender individuals at different stages of the transgender process. However, *de ambiente* is less inclusive than the MSM category, because it refers to individuals who have some connection between their sexual behavior and their self-identification. That is, unlike heterosexually identified MSM, *de ambiente* men are individuals who fall in love with one another, sustain long-term romantic relations with each other, and struggle with the fact that their homosexual behavior is a central aspect of their identities and lives in a society hostile towards homosexuality. In other words, those who are *de ambiente* are self-identified, but not necessarily publicly so to other segments of society.

The outreach card capitalizes on Latino values about the importance of family and was designed to address the need for a "peer family" in men who feel very disconnected from their own families. That is why, on the back side of the card, we present our program meetings as events that resemble dinner time at a family gathering. The card says "dinner is already served *(la cena ya está servida)* and the only thing that is missing is that you join us in our conversation" *(y solo falta que tu te incorpores a nuestras conversaciones)*. Only then, we tell participants that it is about a four-meeting program for Latino gay and bisexual men, "where we will exchange opinions about themes that are important to you and me" *(donde se intercambian opiniones sobre temas que a ti y a mi me interesan)*.

Note that the card is personalized by writing it in the first person from a peer perspective, "important to you and me." The fact that the program is run by peers in a friendly atmosphere is further reinforced and personalized by a picture of the program staff—all Latino gay men, including the present author and researcher, who collaborated in the design and implementation of the program. On the picture we inscribed in larger print what we believe is the most important message of social inclusion: "The only thing missing is you" *(Solo faltas tú !!)*.

The card also tells men about the material incentives ($10 per meeting and a t-shirt if they attend the whole cycle) and the fact that dinner will be served at every meeting. The card also gives potential participants a number to call for more information and to enroll themselves in the program.

Group Intervention

Men who enroll in the program participate in a four-session, small-group intervention. Sessions last two hours each and take place on a weekly basis, for a total commitment of four weeks of participation. The groups are facilitated by two Latino gay men who are trained health educators, including myself, and are conducted using the principles of empowerment education (Shor, 1992; Wallerstein and Bernstein, 1994). As suggested by empowerment models of intervention, facilitators do not "transmit" information or resources (unless specifically requested by the participants). Rather, facilitators engage participants in a reflective dialogue that promotes critical thinking and self-observation about matters of crucial importance to the group.

The role of the facilitators is fivefold; namely, they (1) encourage the orderly and fair participation of all members of the group; (2) ask questions that promote critical thinking ; (3) reflect back to the group the major points of convergence in response to the questions asked; (4) respond to the group's questions about specific information and resources; and (5) present to the group factual information (such as documented rates of HIV infection and unprotected intercourse in Latino gay men) to stimulate discussion and elicit the group's reaction to data about their own community. Sessions typically end with questions about possible solutions or potential actions that address (with concrete action) the problems raised by the discussion. The sessions attempt to accomplish the four essential elements of the intervention described above.

Session 1 is devoted to an examination of participants' lives as Latino gay men, including experiences of rejection and abuse for being gay, issues of coming out to family, sources of social support and community, lover and boyfriend relationships, and related hardships of immigration, poverty, and minority status. Facilitators pose open-ended questions such as "What is the most difficult thing about being a gay man in Latino communities?" "Did you ever have problems in school for being gay?" "How has your family reacted to your being gay?" "Who can you talk to about the things that really matter in your life?" The first goal of the session is to promote participants' awareness about the difficulties involved in their dual-minority status—that is, the issues about being gay and bisexual in a homophobic and machista culture, and the issues about being an ethnic minority in a racist society. The second goal is to promote a sense of bonding and community among persons who have experienced similar types of oppression in their lives.

Session 2 is devoted to an in-depth examination of the impact of AIDS in the participants' lives, including their sexuality. Questions include "How has AIDS affected you?" "Have you lost many friends to the epidemic?" "Are there some aspects of AIDS that you feel confused about?" "What changes have you had to make in your life to cope with the epidemic?" "How has AIDS affected your sexual life?" One goal of the second session is to express feelings about the losses involved in the experience of HIV and AIDS, allowing the participants to begin expressing their concerns, struggles, and difficulties with respect to the practice of safer sex. A second goal of the session is to elicit potential areas of confusion regarding means of HIV transmission and modes of prevention that require further information and clarification. A third and final goal of this second session is to engage the participants in dialogue on issues about sexuality and AIDS.

Session 3 is devoted to a systematic examination of the practice of safer sex, including barriers and facilitators, in participants' experience. Through appropriate questions, participants are led to a critical reflection about situations, thoughts, and feelings that might make the practice of safer sex more difficult, including sex under the influence of alcohol and drugs, anonymous sex in public cruising places, and sex within relations of unequal power. Participants are also encouraged to reflect on those situations, thoughts, and feelings that have actually helped them to practice safer sex. During the second half of this session, facilitators rephrase and mirror the group's stated barriers and difficulties. Participants are then asked to react and devise strategies to deal with those barriers and difficulties. A major goal of this group process is to help participants articulate and construct (from within, rather than facilitator-given) strategies that might address the stated barriers and difficulties, including the possibility of avoiding those situations and circumstances that undermine their sense of personal control over sexual behavior.

Session 4 is devoted to training the group in the use of the safer sex journal (described below) and to construct a summary and integration of lessons learned in the group experience. Participants are asked questions such as "What was the most important thing you learned in the group?" "Are there some things you wanted to say or talk about that you did not have time to say?" "What was the most difficult thing for you about the group?" "What would you like to see different?" Toward the end of the session, participants are invited to participate in the ongoing support group, and available services of prevention case management, described below, are explained to them.

Participants are compensated $50 for their participation in the group intervention; $10 is given at the end of each of the first three sessions and $20 at the end of the last session. Those who attend all four sessions also receive a t-shirt with the program's name and logo. In addition, to encourage a sense of solidarity, a relaxed atmosphere, and on-time participation, food is served during the 30 minutes prior to the beginning of each group meeting.

Follow-up Activities

Safer Sex Journal

During the fourth group session, a set of 30 printed 5" x 8" index cards are distributed to participants. The cards are bound with an attractive cover and presented as "the sexual activity journal" or, as both staff and participants have labeled it *"El Diario del Amor"* (The Journal of Love). Each card contains a set of closed- and open-ended questions to be filled out by participants within 24 hours of a sexual encounter. The journal is for the exclusive and confidential use of the participants and is distributed as "a tool to help you understand your sexuality better and make the practice of safer sex a bit easier."

The journal, all in Spanish and developed in collaboration with health educators and Latino gay clients of Mission Neighborhood Health Center, includes the following questions, all answered for a given sexual encounter, and roughly divided into four different sections.

The first section consists of two general questions about the sexual encounter: "How was it for you?" *(Qué tal te fue?),* to be answered on a 1–10 scale from 1—*Awful (Muy Mal)*—to 10—*Fabulous (Fabuloso).* The second question asks: Why? In other words, why was the encounter awful, fabulous, or somewhere in between?

It is interesting to observe men's reactions to this first section. The men seem well-accustomed to talking about their sexual encounters along a continuum from awful to fabulous, or whatever equivalent colorful adjectives they choose to describe them. The ratings of examples of sexual encounters (we elicit those in the group meetings on a volunteer basis in order to train men in the use of the safer sex journal) are typically accompanied by a lot of laughter, as men recall both fun and not-so-fun sexual experiences.

The group's mood typically changes, however, for the second question, Why? Most of the time it seems as if men have never asked themselves that question. They seem both surprised and glad to have the opportunity to reflect about themselves as sexual beings. Many move their eyes indicating deep reflection, as if this was the first time they have answered for themselves explicitly what they like and don't like sexually. Facilitators are encouraged to use this opportunity to communicate the fact that many of us don't seem to know ourselves sexually and connect this lack of self-knowledge to the few opportunities we have to talk or reflect about our sexuality, apart from sexual boasting or gossip about our sexual encounters.

The program staff believe that a social discourse about ourselves as sexual beings must precede any reflection about barriers or difficulties to safer sex. By creating a social dialogue first (in the group) and providing opportunities for private individual self-reflection about sexuality (through the journal), we provide a first entry to the sexual world of participants and, in our view, open up the possibility for sexual self-observation. The social discourse and self-reflection promoted by the safer sex journal thus becomes a first step toward having access to and some understanding of sexual feelings, desires, and behavior. In line with Bandura's ideas about self-observation, our philosophy is that when there is no access or awareness, there is no possible self-regulation. By promoting self-reflection in the sexual domain, this first section of the journal constitutes an important step toward the self-regulation of risky sexual behavior.

The second section of the journal asks men to rate the sexual encounter, on a scale from 1–10, along five different dimensions: *boring-passionate, silent-communicative, cold and distant, affectionate,* and *unprotected-protected.* This second section of the journal gives men five different windows to observe and examine a sexual encounter, including its safety vis-à-vis HIV transmission.

By including safety as *one* of the many dimensions of a sexual encounter, and particularly as a dimension that is independent from passion, we try to convey two important notions to the participants. First, we want to communicate the fact that safety, affection, and, more importantly, passion can co-exist in a sexual encounter. Second, we want to convey the notion that safety vis-à-vis HIV transmission is neither a black-and-white issue nor a dichotomous safe-unsafe dimension. Rather, we communicate that a sexual encounter can be made increasingly safer through different actions and conditions. We believe that the rigid notion that sex is either safe or unsafe promotes a definition of safe sex as an external standard or guideline that must be followed, and does not open much room for men to act as self-regulating agents in sexual encounters. The perception of sexual safety as a continuous rather than a dichotomous variable, in our view, communicates the notion that sexual episodes can be made increasingly safer through participants' choices and actions.

The third section of the journal is designed to promote a systematic reflection of contextual or person-situation factors that either compete with or facilitate the enactment of safer sex intentions. We accomplish this by presenting side-by-side two different columns. The left column is labeled "What helped you protect yourself" *(Te ayudó a protegerte)* and the right column is labeled "What did *not* help you protect yourself" *(No ayudó a protegerte).* Under each column there are four different categories: thoughts, emotions, situation, and other/partner. Three empty lines under each category are provided for men to fill in their responses.

We encourage men to think about a given situation and examine what helped them and what didn't help them be safe. If possible, we ask for a volunteer to share a sexual event "where it was difficult to practice safer sex." Note that by promoting a reflection of both barriers and facilitators, we present the enactment of safer sex as involving some degree of difficulty or struggle on the part of the sexual agent. The "struggle" involves dealing with potential competing factors that could be of a cognitive, affective, situational, or interpersonal nature. This presentation of safer sex, as not a virtue of "good boys" but as a struggle (at times heroic) of men trying to live full sexual lives in the midst of a devastating epidemic opens up the possibility of a non-punitive dialogue about slips into unsafe practices, while maintaining safer sex as the desirable group norm.

An open and non-punitive discourse about unsafe sex is, in our opinion, one of the most crucial elements of the program's success. We believe that programs that promote safer sex as the group norm, in a rigid and unidimensional way, run the risk of inhibiting or driving underground any meaningful communication about risky sex. If we inhibit the social discourse about risky sexual activity, we undermine one of the most important goals of our program, that is, the critical reflection and observation of person-situation contexts that affect our ability to enact safer sex intentions. The presentation of safer sex as a "struggle" with both barriers and facilitators allows *both* the establishment of the social norm as well as the critical examination of unsafe practices in our lives.

Finally, in the fourth section of the journal we ask men a provocative question: "What would you do different next time?" *(Qué harías diferente la próxima vez?).* The question is designed to promote the construction and development of strategies that could counteract the competing factors and, above all, to open up a window of self-efficacy in situations where men have perceived themselves as helpless. We believe, and have witnessed in the context of the safer sex journal, that hopelessness and helplessness, the converse of self-efficacy, in safer sex can be counteracted by considering the possibilities and imagining scenarios of personal agency in difficult sexual situations.

As readers probably have noticed by now, the safer sex journal is a tool that embodies and contains most of the essential elements of our philosophy for HIV-prevention interventions. The journal is also our main tool to facilitate the transition from social and interpersonal discourse to personal self-observation. The journal is thus a tool to facilitate the internalization of the program's group experience.

Ongoing Peer Support Group

A fortunate problem encountered at the early stages of the program's implementation was the fact that many "graduates" of the four-week cycle wanted to maintain their connection to the program, and many of them simply refused to disengage and continued to show up in subsequent meeting cycles. We quickly realized that graduates needed an ongoing group to continue both the social-support relationships they had developed in the course of the four-week program and also to continue the type of "different" conversations they had encountered with us. The different conversations referred to the process of self-observation and critical self-reflection about their lives they had so immensely enjoyed in the context of our program. This overwhelming enthusiasm for the program surprised many of us who had heard time and time again from HIV service providers the unjustified complaint that Latinos are hard to recruit and that they don't show up to small-group meeting, and so forth. (I am now convinced that those complaints and criticisms apply mostly to the types of programs offered rather than to potential participants).

We then started an ongoing support group for graduates of the four-week cycle. Graduates are encouraged to attend whenever they feel they want contact with the group; they know the suport group is available on a weekly basis for their attendance any time they want or need to. With the help of a staff facilitator, members of the ongoing support group select the topics they want to talk about. Topics selected have included romantic relationships, domestic violence between gay men, drug and alcohol use, and immigration issues, to name a few. Facilitators follow the same principles of empowerment education in the facilitation of group process and discussions.

Monthly Meetings

In order to encourage further a sense of belonging to the program, participants and their partners and friends are invited to monthly meetings of HLS. Monthly meetings are held the week after the end of a four-meeting cycle. The evening of the monthly meeting, both the new cohort of graduates and members of the ongoing social support group as well as their invited guests attend. Monthly meetings consist of talks by invited speakers, video presentations, raffles, group discussion, and participatory activities and games. These meetings serve three important objectives. First, they provide an opportunity to invite potential participants who are curious about the group and want to check out the program before enrolling themselves in a four-week cycle. Second, the monthly meeting serves as a stepping stone between the four-week cycle and the ongoing support group. During the monthly meetings, we ask members of the ongoing support group to tell new graduates about it, and we also ask new graduates to speak about their experiences in their four-week cycle. This exchange between new graduates and long-term members keeps the group refreshed with new ideas and enthusiasm as new cohorts of participants join the follow-up activities and the general brotherhood of HLS.

Finally, the monthly meetings provide an excellent opportunity for staff or invited speakers to do presentations that follow a more didactic, knowledge-transmission-oriented pedagogy. By having the more didactic sessions limited to the monthly meetings, we avoid the staff's temptation to be more didactic during the ongoing meetings, and at the same time provide important information that is either explicitly requested by members or suggested by members' questions and expressed sources of confusion.

Prevention Case Management

The third component of our follow-up activities offers the services of prevention case managers who act as individual counselors or safer sex mentors to program participants, and specifically to those who, in the staff's judgment, could benefit from such services. Prevention case management is particularly encouraged for those individuals who express serious barriers to safer sex and those who have other related needs such as mental health or substance abuse problems. In fact, all participants are encouraged to contact case managers on the phone, or face-to-face, if they feel they need to discuss personal issues in an individual one-to-one session.

The main purpose of prevention case management is to assist program participants in remaining HIV negative or in reducing the risk of re-infection with HIV. This is typically accomplished by identifying the issues that put the individual at risk, and developing a plan to address those issues. Participants are encouraged to discuss with the case manager the results of their sexual activity journaling and any other concerns or difficulties they are encountering in maintaining safer sex practices over time. Based on these data and further assessments of risk, prevention case managers, under the supervision of clinical staff at the Mission Neighborhood Health Center, develop an individualized treatment plan, contract for a given number of sessions, and track referrals for other services and the outcome of those referrals.

In our experience to date, approximately 10% of the participants of HLS have signed up for prevention case management services. Beyond the one-to-one counseling sessions, participants who have attended prevention case management have benefited from a number of other related services such as referrals to substance abuse programs in the city, connection to HIV testing and counseling, and enrollment in clinical trials for the aggressive treatment of acute infection due to recent exposure to HIV.

Program Evaluation

Thus far, the program *Hermanos de Luna y Sol* has been evaluated in terms of its implementation and clients' perceptions of program effects. In what follows, I would like to present very succinctly the data we have regarding the program's ability to attract participants that are often considered "hard to reach" and also participants' evaluations of the effect of the program on factors relevant to HIV prevention in their lives. The intervention is currently in place and running; the present evaluation data covers approximately one year of the program's activities, from its beginning in May 1995 through June 1996.

Program Implementation

As of June 1996, a total of 217 outreach and recruitment interviews were conducted at several Latino-identified gay bars in San Francisco's Mission district. The outreach interviews lasted approximately 10 minutes each and revealed important facts for the target population. The overwhelming majority of the men interviewed at the bars stated that there is no place, other than gay bars, for Latino gay men to gather and talk about important issues in their lives. Similarly, men stated that HIV is very high on their list of worries and concerns. In connection with the recruitment and outreach activities, approximately 2,000 program cards were distributed across different gay venues in the Mission district.

As a result of our outreach and recruitment activities, we were able to enroll 245 individuals into the program; of those, 122 (or 50%) participated at least once in the program. A 50% participation rate represents a decline from the 75% participation obtained during the first six months of the program. The decline might be due to the fact that at the beginning of the program we recruited the most highly motivated individuals in the target population. Men who enrolled later as a result of our outreach and recruitment activities might be less motivated to participate in HIV-prevention interventions. This finding suggests that, in order to sustain the program over time at relatively high levels of enrollment and participation, it is important to maintain the program's outreach and recruitment component at the highest possible level of effort.

By June 25, 1996, a total of 122 different men had attended our group intervention. Of those, 87 (or 71%) attended multiple sessions. The majority of participants were between the ages of 20 and 40, with some representation of men in their 40s. We engaged participants from the following age groups: under 20 = 3 (or 2%); in their 20s = 45 (or 37%); in their 30s = 46 (or 38%); and 40 and above = 28 (or 23%). Ninety-eight participants (or 80%) were born outside the U.S., with the following reported places of birth: Mexico, 61; the Caribbean, 14;

Central America, 14; and South America, 9. The overwhelming majority of participants—102 (or 84%)—identified themselves as gay and homosexual; 16 (or 13%) participants identified themselves as bisexual, and 4 (or 3%) participants identified themselves as transsexual.

During the first year of the program, we completed a total of nine small-group meeting cycles: eight cycles of *four* two-hour weekly meetings each and one cycle of *six* two-hour weekly meetings. We decided to increase the length of the small-group meeting cycles from four to six weeks, only on an experimental basis, and it is still too early to tell whether it shows improved effectiveness. However, our one six-meeting cycle suggested that six meetings is a better number of sessions to implement all the activities proposed and achieve our desired goals.

In-between the small-group meeting cycles, we held eight monthly meetings *(Encuentro Mensual)* that had an average attendance of 22 men per meeting, with the number of participants ranging from 14 to 36. The monthly meetings have been very successful in transitioning the new members to the ongoing support group and in fostering the program's role as a source of social support for all graduates of the program. We have used the monthly meetings to bring in speakers from different agencies servicing Latino gay men in the area and to provide requested instruction on topics of interest to program participants. For example, we have hosted invited speakers on nutrition, on HIV testing, on services for HIV-positive individuals, on volunteering, and on immigration issues. Above all, the monthly meetings have created an atmosphere of social support and enjoyment, and these have helped us bring back some graduates of the program who have been out of touch for a while. We also have invited to the monthly meetings the new enrollees so they can meet other participants before they begin their small-group meeting cycle.

During the first year of the program, we had a total of 24 weekly meetings of the ongoing social-support group. The average attendance of participants to this component of the program was 8 per group meeting, with the number of participants ranging from 5 to 15. Participants have selected the topics of discussion, including relationships, experiences of sexual abuse, relations to family, and coming-out issues for Latinos, to name a few.

Participants' Perceptions of Program Effects

At the end of each four-week cycle, we have asked participants to state their responses to seven questions regarding the impact of the group meetings on different aspects of their lives related to the goals of the program. In what follows, I list the results of the tabulated responses for 78 group participants.

HAS THE GROUP HELPED YOU TO . . .

1. FEEL MORE CONNECTED TO THE LATINO GAY COMMUNITY?

0%	17%	36%	47%
NOT AT ALL	A BIT	SUBSTANTIALLY	A LOT

2. FEEL BETTER ABOUT YOURSELF?

0%	15%	49%	36%
NOT AT ALL	A BIT	SUBSTANTIALLY	A LOT

3. BETTER UNDERSTAND YOUR SEXUALITY?

4%	21%	41%	34%
NOT AT ALL	A BIT	SUBSTANTIALLY	A LOT

4. REFLECT ON YOUR OWN RISK FOR HIV?

0%	13%	46%	41%
NOT AT ALL	A BIT	SUBSTANTIALLY	A LOT

5. FEEL MORE CAPABLE TO PRACTICE SAFER SEX?

1%	11%	45%	43%
NOT AT ALL	A BIT	SUBSTANTIALLY	A LOT

6. REAFFIRM YOUR INTENTION TO PRACTICE SAFER SEX?

0%	12%	35%	53%
NOT AT ALL	A BIT	SUBSTANTIALLY	A LOT

7. AVOID SITUATIONS THAT ARE DIFFICULT TO PRACTICE SAFER SEX?

0%	13%	41%	45%
NOT AT ALL	A BIT	SUBSTANTIALLY	A LOT

As can be seen from the above results, the majority of participants felt that the intervention had a strong impact on different aspects of their lives. Interestingly, the effect was especially strong for items related to HIV and safer sex. Participants' responses suggest that group meetings are especially helpful to (1) reaffirm their intentions to practice safer sex (item 6); (2) increase their self-efficacy to practice safer sex (item 5) ; and (3) avoid situations that are difficult to practice safer sex (item 7). In addition, participants strongly agreed that the program makes them feel more connected to the Latino gay community (item 1).

To date, we have only piloted the possibility of a pre-post-evaluation of the program's effects on behavioral outcomes. We have had some difficulty in tracking participants over time for four-month follow-up (post-test) interviews. However, beginning in January 1997 with recently obtained funds, we will conduct an evaluation of behavioral outcomes that includes moderately aggressive efforts to track participants over time. Unfortunately, as of this writing, I do not have the data to comment on the effectiveness of the HLS program to affect the incidence of HIV risk behavior.

Nonetheless, results of the survey on participants' perceptions are highly encouraging. The fact that participants gave the highest endorsement to items directly related to HIV prevention confirms our belief that by addressing the cultural context that promotes risk, even in the absence of an intensive and directive campaign to use condoms, Latino gay men will reaffirm their intentions and commitment to practice safer sex.

The findings to date provide some support for one of the main ideas of the present book. Namely, by promoting critical self-observation on the sociocultural factors that regulate our sexuality, Latino gay men will increase their sense of self-efficacy in the practice of safer sex.

References

Almaguer, T. (1991). Chicano men: A cartography of homosexual identity and behavior. *Differences: A Journal of Feminist Cultural Studies, 3*(2), 75–100.

Amaro, H. (1995). Love, sex and power: Considering women's realities in HIV prevention. *American Psychologist, 50,* 437–447.

Amaro, H., and Gornermann, I. (1992). *HIV/AIDS related knowledge, attitudes beliefs and behaviors among Hispanics in the Northeast and Puerto Rico: Report of findings and recommendations.* Paper presented at the Northeast Hispanic AIDS Consortium, Boston University School of Public Health, Boston, MA.

Bandura, A. (1986). *Social foundations of thought and action: A social cognitive theory.* Englewood Cliffs, NJ: Prentice-Hall.

Bandura, A. (1994). Social cognitive theory and exercise of control over HIV infection. In R. J. DiClemente and J. L. Peterson (Eds.), *Preventing AIDS: Theories and methods of behavioral interventions* (pp. 25–59). New York: Plenum Press.

Baumeister, L., Flores, E., and Marín, B. (1995). Sex information given to Latina adolescents by parents. *Health Education Research, 10*(2), 233–239.

Baumrind, D. (1985). Familial antecedents of adolescent drug use: A developmental perspective. In C. L. Jones and R. J. Battjes (Eds.), *Etiology of adolescent drug abuse: Implications for prevention. NIDA Research Monograph* (Vol. 56). Rockville, MD: National Institute on Drug Abuse.

Carballo-Diéguez, A. (1989). Hispanic culture, gay male culture, and AIDS: Counseling implications. *Journal of Counseling and Development, 68,* 26–30.

Carballo-Diéguez, A. (1995). Sexual HIV-risk behavior among Puerto Rican men who have sex with men. In G. M. Herek and B. Greene (Eds.), *AIDS and the Lesbian and Gay Community.* Thousand Oaks, CA: SAGE.

Carballo-Diéguez, A., and Dolezal, C. (1995). Association between history of childhood sexual abuse and adult HIV-risk sexual behavior in Puerto Rican men who have sex with men. *Child Abuse and Neglect, 19*(5), 595–605.

Carrier, J. (1989). Gay liberation and coming out in Mexico. *Journal of Homosexuality, Special Issue: Gay and Lesbian Youth II, 17*(3–4), 225–252.

Catania, J., Coates, T., and Stall, R. (1991). Changes in condom use among homosexual men in San Francisco. *Health Psychology, 10*(3), 190–199.

Catania, J. A., Kegeles, S. M., and Coates, T. J. (1990). Towards an understanding of risk behavior: An AIDS Risk Reduction Model (ARRM). *Health Education Quarterly, 17*(1), 53–72.

CDC (1991). Characteristics of parents who discuss AIDS with their children—United States, 1989. *MMWR, 22*(40), 789–791.

CDC (1993a). *HIV/AIDS Surveillance Report, Year-end Edition: U.S. AIDS cases reported through December, 1992.* Atlanta, GA: Centers for Disease Control and Prevention.

CDC (1993b). *HIV/AIDS Surveillance Report, First Quarter Edition* (5[1]). Atlanta, GA: Centers for Disease Control and Prevention.

CDC (1994). *HIV/AIDS Surveillance Report* (6[1], pp. 1–27). Atlanta, GA: Centers for Disease Control and Prevention.

CDC (1996). *HIV/AIDS Surveillance Report* (8[1]). Atlanta, GA: Centers for Disease Control.

Ceballos-Capitaine, A., Szapocznik, J., Blaney, N. T., Morgan, R. O., Millon, C., and Eisdorfer, C. (1990). Ethnicity, emotional distress, stress-related disruption, and coping among HIV seropositive gay males. *Hispanic Journal of Behavioral Sciences, 12*(2), 135–152.

Coates, T. J., Stall, R. D., Catania, J. A., and Kegeles, S. (1988). Behavioral factors in HIV infection. *AIDS, 2 (Suppl.1)*, S239–S246.

Day, S., and Ward, H. (1990). The Praed Street Project: A cohort of prostitute women in London. In M. Plant (Ed.), *AIDS, Drugs and Prostitution.* London: Routledge.

Deci, E. L., and Ryan, R. M. (1985). *Intrinsic motivation and self-determination in human behavior.* New York: Plenum Press.

Díaz, R. M., Morales, E., Dilán, E., and Rodríguez, R. (n.d.). *Demographic, developmental, and psychosocial correlates of risky sexual behavior among Latino gay men in San Francisco.*Unpublished manuscript.

Díaz, R. M., Neal, C. J. and Amaya-Williams, M. (1990). The social origins of self-regulation. In L. C. Moll (Ed.), *Vygotsky and education: Instructional implications and applications of sociohistorical psychology* (pp. 127–154). New York: Cambridge University Press.

Díaz, R. M., Stall, R. D., Hoff, C., Daigle, D., and Coates, T. J. (1996). HIV Risk Among Latino Gay Men in the Southwestern United States. *AIDS Education and Prevention, 8*(5), 415–429.

Doll, L. S., Byers, R. H., Bolan, G., Douglas, J. M., Moss, P. M., Weller, P. D., Joy, D., Bartholow, B. N., and Harrison, J. S. (1991). Homosexual men who engage in high risk behavior: A multicenter comparison. *Sexually Transmitted Diseases, 18*(3), 170–175.

Enchautegui, M. E. (1995). *Policy implications of Latino poverty.* Washington, DC: The Urban Institute.

Fairbank, B., and Maullin, Inc. (1991). *A survey of AIDS knowledge, attitudes and behaviors in San Francisco's American-Indian, Filipino and Latino gay and bisexual males communities.* San Francisco: San Francisco Department of Public Health, AIDS Office.

Ferriss, S. (1993). Fatalismo: A health threat for Latinos. *San Francisco Examiner,* January 19, pp. A1–A14.

Fishbein, M., Bandura, A., Triandis, H. C., Kanfer, F. H., and Becker, M. H. (1991). *Factors influencing behavior and behavior change: Final report—Theorists' Workshop.* Washington, DC: National Institute of Mental Health.

Fisher, J. D., Fisher, W. A., Williams, S. S., and Malloy, T. E. (1994). Empirical tests of an information-motivation-behavioral skills model of AIDS-preventive behavior with gay men and heterosexual university students. *Health Psychology, 13,* 238–250.

Freire, P. (1993). *Education for critical consciousness.* New York: Seabury.

Gagnon, J., and Simon, W. (1973). *Sexual conduct: The social sources of human sexuality.* Illinois: Adine.

García-Coll, C. (1990). Developmental outcome of minority infants: A process-oriented look into our beginnings. *Child Development, 61,* 270–289.

Helman, C. (1990). *Culture, health and illness.* Oxford: Butterworth-Heinemann.

Hoffman, M. L. (1970). Moral development. In P. H. Mussen (Ed.), *Carmichael's Handbook of Child Psychology* (Vol. 2). New York: Wiley.

Keesing, R. M. (1981). *Cultural anthropology: A contemporary perspective.* New York: Holt, Rinehart and Winston.

Kegeles, S. M., Hays, R. B., and Coates, T. J. (1996). The Empowerment project: A community-level HIV prevention intervention for young gay men. *American Journal of Public Health, 86*(8).

Kelley, P., Miller, R., Pomerantz, R., Wann, F., Brundage, J., and Burke, D. (1990). Human immunodeficiency virus and seropositivity among members of the active duty U.S. Army 1985–1989. *American Journal of Public Health, 80*(4), 405–410.

Kelly, J. A., Kalichman, S. C., Kauth, M. R., Kilgore, H. G., Hood, H. V., Campos, P. E., Rao, S. M., Brasfield, T. L., and St. Lawrence, J. S. (1991). Situational factors associated with AIDS risk behavior lapses and coping strategies used by gay men who successfully avoid lapses. *American Journal of Public Health, 81*(10), 1335–1338.

Kimmel, M. (1995). *Manhood in America: A cultural analysis.* New York: Free Press.

Kingsley, L. A. (1991). Temporal trends in Human Immunodeficiency Virus Type 1 Seroconversion 1984–1989: A Report from the Multicenter AIDS Cohort Study (MACS). *American Journal of Epidemiology, 134*(4), 331–339.

Kochems, L. M. (1987). *Meanings and health implications: Gay men's sexuality.* Paper presented at the American Anthropological Association.

Kuhl, J., and Beckmann, J. (Eds.). (1985). *Action control: From cognition to behavior.* New York: Springer-Verlag.

Kupers, T. A. (1995). What do men want? *Readings: A Journal of Reviews and Commentary in Mental Health, 10*(4), 16–21.

LaFramboise, T., Coleman, H., and Gerton, J. (1993). Psychological impact of biculturalism: Evidence and theory. *Psychological Bulletin, 114*(3), 395–412.

Lemp, G. (1994). Seroprevalence of HIV and risk behaviors among young homosexual and bisexual men: The San Francisco/Berkeley young men's survey. *Journal of the American Medical Association*, *272*, 449–454.

Leviton, L. C. (1989). Theoretical foundations of AIDS-prevention programs. In R. O. Valdiserri (Ed.), *Preventing AIDS: The design of effective programs*. New Brunswick, NJ: Rutgers University Press.

Lindan, C., Hearst, N., Singleton, J., Trachtenberg, A., Riordan, N., Tokagawa, D., and Chu, G. (1990). Underreporting of Minority AIDS Deaths in San Francisco Bay Area, 1985–1986. *Public Health Reports, 105*(4), 400–404.

Lumsden, I. (1991). *Homosexuality, society and the state in Mexico*. Mexico, DF: Solediciones, Colectivo Sol.

Marín, B. V., Tschann, J., and Gómez, C. (1993). Multiple heterosexual partners and condom use among Hispanics and non-Hispanic whites. *Public Health Reports, 108*(6), 742–750.

Marín, G., and Marín, B. V. (1991). *Research with Hispanic populations*. Newbury Park, CA: Sage.

NCA. (1992). *The challenge of HIV/AIDS in communities of color*. Washington, DC: National Commission on AIDS.

NTFAP. (1993). *The 1991 Southern States AIDS Education Survey: A knowledge, attitudes and behavior study of African-American, Latino, and White men, Final Report*. San Francisco: National Task Force on AIDS Prevention.

Osmond, D. H., Page, K., Wiley, J., Garrett, K., Sheppard, H. W., Moss, A. R., Schrager, L., and Winkelstein, W. (1994). HIV infection in homosexual and bisexual men 18–29 years of age: The San Francisco young men's health study. *American Journal of Public Health, 84*, 1933–1937.

Padilla, A. M. (1980). *Acculturation: Theory, models and some new findings*. Boulder, CO: Westview.

Padilla, E. (1987). Sexuality among Mexican-Americans: A case of sexual stereotyping. *Journal of Personality and Social Psychology, 52*, 5–10.

Pérez-Stable, E. J., Sabogal, F., and Otero-Sabogal, R. (1995). Use of cancer screening tests in the San Francisco Bay Area. *Monographs of the National Cancer Institute, 18*, 147–153.

PMC. (1995). *The impact of homophobia and other social biases on AIDS*. San Francisco: Public Media Center.

Prieur, A. (1990). Norwegian gay men: Reasons for continued practice of unsafe sex. *AIDS Education and Prevention*, 2(2), 109–115.

Ramírez, J., Suarez, E., de la Rosa, G., Castro, M. A., and Zimmerman, M. A. (1994). AIDS knowledge and sexual behavior among Mexican gay and bisexual men. *AIDS Education and Prevention*, 6(2), 163–174.

Remien, R. H., Carballo-Diéguez, A., and Wagner, G. (1995). Intimacy and sexual risk behaviour in serodiscordant male couples. *AIDS Care*, 7(4), 429–438.

Richwald, G. A., Morisky, E. E., Kyle, G. R., Kristal, A. R., Gerber, M. M., and Friedland, J. M. (1988). Sexual activities in bathhouses in Los Angeles County: Implications for AIDS prevention education. *The Journal of Sex Research*, 24(2), 169–180.

Rotter, J. B. (1971). External control and internal control. *Psychology Today*, 5(n1, 37–42), 58–59.

Sabogal, F., Marin, G., Otero-Sabogal, R., Marin, B. V., and Perez-Stable, E. (1987). Hispanic familism and acculturation: What changes and what doesn't. *Hispanic Journal of Behavioral Sciences*, 9(4), 397–412.

Sabogal, F., Sandlin, G., Reyes, R., Aguirre, V., Bregman, G., and Lemp, G. (1991). *San Francisco Latino gay/bisexual males' HIV knowledge, attitudes and behaviors*. Paper presented at the American Psychological Association Annual Convention.

Sabogal, F., Sandlin, G., Reyes, R., Aguirre, V., Bregman, G., and Lemp, G. (1992). Hombres Latinos gay y bisexuales: Una comunidad de alto riesgo del VIH/SIDA. [Latino gay and sexual men: A community at high risk for HIV/AIDS.] *Revista Latinoamericana de Psicologia*, 24(1–2), 57–69.

Seibt, A. C., and McAlister, A. L. (1993). Condom use and sexual identity among men who have sex with men. *MMWR*, 42(1), 7–14.

SFDH. (1993). *Estimates of the number of persons infected with HIV in San Francisco by Race/ethnicity*. San Francisco: Surveillance Branch, AIDS Office, San Francisco Department of Public Health.

Shor, I. (1992). *Empowering education: Critical teaching for social change*. Chicago: University of Chicago Press.

Simon, W. (1996). *Postmodern sexualities*. New York: Routledge.

St. Louis, M., Conway, G., Hayman, C., Miller, C., Petersen, L., and Dondero, T. (1991). Human immunodeficiency virus infection in disadvantaged adolescents. *Journal of the American Medical Association, 266*(17), 2387–2391.

Stall, R., Barrett, D., Bye, L., Catania, J., Frutchey, C., Henne, J., Lemp, G., and Paul, J. (1992). A comparison of younger and older gay men's HIV risk-taking behaviors: The communication technologies 1989 cross-sectional survey. *Journal of the Acquired Immune Deficiency Disorders, 5*, 682.

Stigler, J. W., Shweder, R. A., and Herdt, G. (Eds.). (1990). *Cultural psychology: Essays on comparative human development.* New York: Cambridge University Press.

Tylor, E. B. (1871). *Primitive culture: Research into the development of mythology, philosophy, religion, art and customs.* London: John Murray.

Wallerstein, N., and Bernstein, E. (1994). Introduction to community empowerment, participatory education and health. *Health Education Quarterly, 21*(2), 141–148.

Index